MONOGRAPH SERIES OF THE
PSYCHOANALYTIC STUDY OF THE CHILD
NO. 5

MONOGRAPH SERIES OF THE
PSYCHOANALYTIC STUDY OF THE CHILD
NO. 5

Studies in Child Psychoanalysis: Pure and Applied

THE SCIENTIFIC PROCEEDINGS OF THE
20TH ANNIVERSARY CELEBRATIONS OF
THE HAMPSTEAD CHILD-THERAPY COURSE
AND CLINIC

by members of the staff
FOREWORD BY ANNA FREUD

New Haven and London
Yale University Press
1975

THE MONOGRAPH SERIES OF THE PSYCHOANALYTIC STUDY OF THE CHILD

Managing Editors: Ruth S. Eissler, Anna Freud, Marianne Kris, Albert J. Solnit

Associate Editor: Lottie M. Newman

Library of Congress catalog card number: 74-20082
International standard book number: 0-300-0-01817-7

Designed by Sally Sullivan
and set in Baskerville type.
Printed in the United States of America by
The Heffernan Press Inc., Worcester, Mass.

Published in Great Britain, Europe, and Africa by
Yale University Press, Ltd., London.
Distributed in Latin America by Kaiman & Polon,
Inc., New York City; in Australasia and Southeast
Asia by John Wiley & Sons Australasia Pty. Ltd.,
Sydney; in India by UBS Publishers' Distributors Pvt.,
Ltd., Delhi; in Japan by John Weatherhill, Inc., Tokyo.

Contents

Acknowledgments   vii

Foreword by Anna Freud   ix

PART I

1. Developments in Child Psychoanalysis in the
   Last Twenty Years, Pure and Applied: A Vital
   Balance
   ALBERT J. SOLNIT   1

2. The Hampstead Child-Therapy Clinic and Legal
   Education
   JOSEPH GOLDSTEIN   15

PART II

3. Depressive Phenomena in Childhood: Their
   Open and Disguised Manifestations in Analytic
   Treatment
   AGNES BENE   33

4. Some Reflections Arising from the Treatment
   of a Traumatized "Borderline" Child
   SARA ROSENFELD   47

5. A Threat of Irreparable Damage
   MARIA KAWENOKA BERGER   65

6. Some Problems of Diagnosis in Children Presenting
   with Obsessional Symptomatology
   CLIFFORD YORKE, RENATE PUTZEL, AND
   LORE SCHACHT   81

7. Aspects of Self Cathexis in "Mainline" Heroin
Addiction: A Preliminary Report
STANLEY   WISEBERG,   CLIFFORD   YORKE,
AND PATRICIA RADFORD   99

8. The Use of the Profile Schema for the Psychotic Patient
THOMAS FREEMAN   117

9. The Nursery School of the Hampstead Child-
Therapy Clinic
ANNA FREUD   127

10. The Border Between Therapy and Education
ROSE EDGCUMBE   133

11. Sexual Fantasies and Sexual Theories in Childhood
JOSEPH SANDLER   149

Bibliography   163

Program for the 20th Anniversary Celebrations of
the Hampstead Clinic   169

Index   171

Acknowledgments

The arrangements for the celebration were in the hands of Miss Agnes Bene, staff member of the Hampstead Clinic and member of the British Psycho-Analytic Society. She succeeded in pressing all staff members and students into service and, together with the Clinic's Administration, set up a Program Committee for the careful scrutiny of available presentations on subjects of clinical, theoretical, training, and applied interests. Invitations were sent out, with the result that on a weekend in July 1972 we received 292 colleagues from psychoanalytic societies and allied professions, a number far exceeding our expectations.

In the first Opening Address which fell to my part, I expressed above all the Clinic's gratitude to its steadfast supporters: to Miss Helen Ross and Mr. Maxwell Hahn of the Field Foundation, New York, as the true founders of the Clinic and the donors of our first house, No. 12 Maresfield Gardens; to Dr. Kurt R. Eissler, as the untiring and unwavering provider for the new venture's ever-increasing needs; to the late Dr. H. Nunberg, former head of the Psychoanalytic Foundation for Research and Development, New York; the late Mr. and Mrs. Currier of the Taconic Foundation, New York, whose generous grants promoted the Clinic's early growth; to the Ford Foundation, New York; to the Grant Foundation, New York, who through the good offices of Miss Adele Morrison, later Dr. Douglas Bond, have maintained our educational and preventive services from their beginnings; to the Grant Foundation, Andrew Mellon Foundation, New York, and Wolfson Foundation, England, for providing us with study grants; to the New-Land Foundation, New York, for the gift of our second house, No. 21 Maresfield Gardens and for other support; to the Clement Stone Foundation, Chicago, for repeated grants;

to the American Government via the National Institute of Mental Health for eleven years of awards toward our developmental studies; to the Freud Centenary Fund, England, for postgraduate psychoanalytic training and many other purposes.

What I left to the last, though by no means least, were our thanks to the only two donors, actually present in the gathering: Mrs. Lita Hazen of the Lita Hazen Charitable Trust, Beverly Hills, California, to whom we owe our third house, No. 14 Maresfield Gardens, and Mrs. Hazen and Dr. R. R. Greenson of the Foundation for Research in Psychoanalysis, California, who give invaluable support to our diagnostic studies.

Here I also want to thank the members of my staff for the work carried out to make the celebration a successful meeting and express my appreciation to those who worked very hard on their presentations.

ANNA FREUD

ANNA FREUD

Foreword

When the Hampstead Child-Therapy Clinic approached the twentieth year of its existence, the younger members of the staff insisted on a celebration of the date. According to the Clinic's custom, this was to be a scientific, not a social, event —an opportunity to acquaint those who would attend with the direction of work being done in the Clinic's various departments. This monograph contains a selection of the scientific proceedings of this meeting.

The Hampstead Child-Therapy Clinic is a successor to the Hampstead Nurseries, which Dorothy Burlingham and I operated during World War II. Left over from this work, after 1945, were a number of interested workers who, for five years, had had the opportunity to witness the processes of childhood in action. Familiar as they were with the children's manifest behavior, they professed themselves eager to enlarge their knowledge by the observable manifestation to their unconscious motivations. These personal wishes to learn met with an urgent need for child therapists in the official services for children, a need especially acknowledged by the late Dr. Kate Friedlaender, who worked at the time for the Child Guidance Clinics of Sussex, England. Thus, the Hampstead Child-Therapy Course came into being, as a training program for psychoanalytic child therapists, i.e., child analysts, not previously trained in therapy for adults. In fact, this was the initial move toward the present organization, which by now has set itself a fourfold aim: to learn, to treat, to teach, and to apply psychoanalytic knowledge to educational and preventive purposes.

It may be asked whether a new creation of this kind is really necessary in a world where psychoanalytic clinics and psychoanalytic training institutes already abound? I believe our existence is justified, in the first instance, by the need to experiment with a full-time involvement of students in a program extending beyond therapy to psychoanalytic research and application, in contrast to the official institutes' restriction to part-time training in clinical and basic theoretical matters only. But beyond these mere differences in organization and planning, I want to emphasize the importance of a different quality of experience that can be obtained in a clinic geared to childhood. There is indeed a need for a place where analytic studies of human development can be pursued not as an adjunct to the analytic therapy of adults but as a main subject in its own right. While it is true that the analysts of adults also are concerned with their patients' infantile prehistory, there remains the fact that they can approach this only via regression, reconstructed from the revival of repressed past experience and selected according to its impact on pathology. In contrast, the child analyst meets the same processes while they are in progress, unselected, and including the transitory upheavals which, while development proceeds, are apt to disappear again without leaving remnants. As child analysts, we thus acquire a view of average, so-called normal, development as the background against which infantile psychopathology can be assessed, while as analysts of adults our glimpses of normality are always seen through and against the background of psychopathological manifestations.

A children's clinic such as ours deals with a range of material different from the intake of the ordinary psychoanalytic clinics. As regards the latter, we are proud enough of the widening scope of psychoanalytic therapy and understanding, both of which by now reach from the neuroses proper to the character disorders and from there to the perversions, delinquencies, and psychotic states. But there is an even wider scope in a children's clinic. It includes the many possible variations of personality development; the atypical personalities caused by deviations in physical or mental endowment and/or deviations in environmental influence; the delays and arrests in growth on any level of drive or ego development or any of the combined developmental lines; the transitory upsèts tied to each developmental stage; the prestructural, quasineurotic disorders caused by conflicts between instinctual wishes and their environmental prohibition; the infantile neuroses caused by conflicts within the internal structure; the borderline, psychosomatic, autistic and psychotic states.

We found that not all the pathological manifestations within this range respond to the psychoanalytic technique as the method of choice, which it is for the neuroses. This experience engendered an interest not shared traditionally by the analysts of adults, namely, an involvement with diagnosis preceding therapy. To further this aim, we set up our Diagnostic Profile, as a metapsychological picture of the child under investigation; a series of Developmental Lines to assess the individual child's developmental status so far as id-ego interaction is concerned; a set of new Diagnostic Categories, based not on psychiatric but on developmental viewpoints; and a new classification of infantile symptomatology based not on phenomenology but on the underlying processes.

Plans of this nature are well beyond any individual's effort; they needed to be assigned to a team of workers. When this happened, findings were pooled and subsequently laid down in the Clinic's Index, a communal memory for classifying and storing psychoanalytic material under analytically meaningful headings and categories. Understandably, such group work depends for its success on the availability of a common scientific language. This need, in its turn, led to the scrutinizing and clarifying of analytic terms and concepts—to work carried out by the Index Department and helped by our Concept Study Groups.

As regards the Clinic's position concerning the technique of child analysis, we do not share the rather widespread ambition that this needs to be identical with the technique for adult analysis in all essential respects. We agree that this identity is valid so far as the patients' id content is concerned. But we see far-reaching differences between the adult's ego, which enters into a treatment alliance with the analyst, and the various levels and stages of the infantile ego which confront the child analyst. It seems to us that it is this developmental level of ego functioning which the technique of child analysis has to take into account, and to which it needs to be adapted to do justice to the child patient. Evidence of this technique in use was offered in several of our clinical case presentations.

The actual program of the Clinic's meeting was organized to reflect the work carried out in all departments. Yet, when it came to publication, a selection had to be made for considerations of space and for other reasons. Thus, this monograph gives no account of our follow-up work of some of our war babies; of the simultaneous analyses of parents and children and the conclusions drawn from them; of our endeavors in the applied field, especially work with pediatricians' groups and interdisciplinary hospital personnel. Equally significant are the omissions concerning the activities of the Nursery School for the Blind and a picture of our training activities, seen from the teachers' as well as from the students' point of view. Much of this is left for future publications.

Part I of the Monograph contains two papers which, as opening addresses, deal with the impact of the Clinic's thought on the Child Study Center of Yale University and the Yale Law school. The papers in Part II are restricted to activities carried out on our own premises.

PART I

ALBERT J. SOLNIT, M.D.

Developments in Child Psychoanalysis in the Last Twenty Years, Pure and Applied: A Vital Balance

Long before the first contacts between the Hampstead Clinic and Yale's Child Study Center, we had known about the Hampstead Nurseries, 1940–1945, through reading and discussing *War and Children* and *Infants Without Families* (A. Freud and Burlingham, 1942–43). Also, Edith Jackson had modestly told us of one aspect of the Vienna phase of institutional development when she described an experimental nursery for children between one and two years of age. We were impressed then, as we are now, that the Anna Freud-Dorothy Burlingham child psychoanalytic group always was flexible and vigorous enough to provide urgently needed services for children and to use these for systematic observations organized by psychoanalytic assumptions. Reexamination of these assumptions usually led to new theoretical questions, refinement of psychoanalytic theory, and the stimulation of further psychoanalytic work. Humanitarian values and passionate scientific inquiry were combined, often without the benefit of financial support for the research aspect of the work in the pre-Hampstead Clinic days.

It is difficult to separate the individual beginnings from the institutional developments. Anna Freud, in her Acknowledg-

Sterling Professor of Pediatrics and Psychiatry and Director, Child Study Center, Yale University; Faculty, Western New England Institute for Psychoanalysis, New Haven, Conn.

1

ments to Volume IV of her *Writings* (1968), has put these
linkages into perspective. She said:

> The majority of papers in this volume owe their existence to
> the author's extension of activities from private practice to
> clinic practice with children, a step which was made possible
> by the creation of The Hampstead Child-Therapy Course
> and Clinic. This organization, an heir to the Hampstead
> Wartime Nurseries, has set itself a fourfold task: to apply
> psychoanalytic therapy to disturbed children of all ages; to
> apply psychoanalytic thinking to the upbringing of normal
> and handicapped children; to increase the body of knowl-
> edge known as psychoanalytic child psychology; to train
> nonmedical candidates in the technique of child analysis,
> child guidance, parent guidance, and the diagnosis of child-
> hood disturbances [p. xv].

The Hampstead Clinic has maintained the tradition of
courageous exploration while becoming an institution of higher
learning with the highest values of education, scholarship, and
service.

Further background for the development of the Hampstead
Clinic and the impact of its work on those concerned with
children throughout the United States, Europe, and Israel was
provided by Anna Freud's introduction to "Observations on
Child Development" (1951):

> For the psychoanalyst who deals habitually with latent, re-
> pressed, and unconscious material, which has to be drawn
> into consciousness by the laborious means of analytic tech-
> nique, a shift of interest to the observation of manifest, overt
> behavior marks a step which is not undertaken without
> misgivings. As psychoanalysts we are not interested in be-
> havioristic data for their own sake. We ask ourselves whether
> observational work outside of the analytic setting can ever
> lead to new discoveries about underlying trends and proces-
> ses, and can thereby supplement the data gathered through
> the analyses of adults and children. *It is therefore helpful to be
> reminded that the origin of our analytic knowledge of children is not
> as exclusively centered in the analytic situation between analyst and*

patient as we are sometimes inclined to believe. It is true that the
basic data concerning the phases of libido development and
the oedipus and castration complexes were extracted during
the psychoanalytic exploration of normal, neurotic or
psychotic adults and children, i.e., with the help of the
analytic technique of free association, and the interpretation
of dreams and transference manifestations. But in later
stages many data were added to this body of knowledge
which came from sources less purely analytic. When the
knowledge concerning infantile sexuality and its transforma-
tions had spread in the circle of psychoanalytic workers,
direct observation of children began. Such observations were
carried out first by parents, either under analysis or analysts
themselves, on their own children, and were recorded regularly in special columns of the psychoanalytic journals of the
time. When psychoanalysis began to be applied to the upbringing of children, the analysis of teachers and nursery
school workers became a frequent occurrence. The observational work of these, professionally trained, people had the
advantage of being undertaken with greater objectivity and
more emotional detachment than parents can muster when
confronted with the behavior of their own children. It had
the further advantage of dealing not only with individuals
but with groups. An additional source of information was
opened up when psychoanalysis began to be applied, not
only to normal educational work, but to work with delinquent and criminal children, and when, again, workers in
this field were analyzed, trained, supervised, and encouraged
to observe. It was the common characteristic of all these
classes of investigators that their observation work was done
on the basis of their personal analyses and their analytic
training and that it was linked with practical activities with
children (upbringing, teaching, therapy). The results helped
to swell the body of existing analytic knowledge, even
though, as Ernst Kris maintains, they did not break new
ground.

[Anna Freud added,] For the analyst who derives his
conviction of the validity of the analytic findings from applying the miscroscope of the psychoanalytic technique, *it is an*

*exciting experience to work for once with the naked eye and to
discover how far the happenings in the deeper layers are actually
reflected in behavior—if one looks for them.* On the other hand,
when assessing the value of such work which can be called
neither analytic nor purely observational, it will be necessary
to keep its limitations in both directions fully in mind [pp.
144f., 148; italics added].

In these lucid descriptions of the methods of care and study
employed in the early experiments in Vienna and by the staff
and leadership of the wartime Hampstead Nurseries there are
significant allusions to a large number of scientific and historical issues. Of the many that come to mind, a number have
already been rediscovered, including:

(a) the development of sustained early interventions for the
deprived young children of low-income, minority or immigrant families;
(b) the urgent need to provide training and supervision for
paraprofessionals in order to avoid the temptation to
offer poor care for poor children;
(c) the careful planning for day-care programs of high quality when the mother cannot stay home during the child's
first three to four years of life;
(d) the recognition that the physically handicapped child can
be helped to master developmental tasks if his potential
psychological capacities are safeguarded through adequate maternal care and early specialized education.

New problems include those of the changing aspects of the
adolescent experience and the increased dependency on and
misuse of drugs.

It has become increasingly clear, as demonstrated by the
work of the Hampstead Child-Therapy Course and Clinic, that
the growth of child psychoanalysis hinges on the interdepen-
dence of psychoanalytic research and its applications. Each
stimulates and refines the other. Just as Ernst Kris (1947) spoke
of the spurious character of a division between "academic" and
"psychoanalytic," I wish to indicate the artificial quality of a
barrier between studies of child development based on the

psychoanalytic treatment (the microscope of psychoanalytic technique) of children, and the studies of children based on direct observation (the macroscope of direct observation). These two approaches are essential and mutually dependent in the study of the developing child.

Anna Freud and Ernst Kris have emphasized the risk of using direct observations to make inferences about underlying mental processes and trends. On the other hand, they have also pointed out that certain kinds of observation, data in given contexts, are available only outside the psychoanalytic treatment situation. For example, much of the data about patterns of close mother-child interaction can be obtained only in action research—research carried out while the observer is supplying a needed intervention as a trusted, helping person. The field of observation is contaminated further by the care, guidance, and support provided by the participant observer, but the data gathered usually are not available to an outsider, a nonparticipant observer.

Direct observations by participating and nonparticipating observers are as essential for our studies as are the psychoanalytic treatment data. The real question, therefore, is how to minimize the distortions by taking into account the limitations of the observations created by the action research, while maintaining a balance between "microscopic" and "macroscopic" studies.

It is crucial to maintain this vital balance in order for child psychoanalysis to maintain an openness to new data, new hypotheses, and the selective and refined rediscovery of the old assumptions and formulations. However, in moving back and forth between the psychoanalytic treatment data and direct observational studies, there is an expected risk: that there will be a loss of definition and a blurring of levels of inference and generalization that each set of studies is capable of producing.

To guard against this risk it is crucial to maintain a critical mass of research based on the psychoanalytic treatment method. Without this "magnification" and sharpening of the microscopic focus there is a strong tendency to rewrite theory by semantic diffusion and the glossing over of theoretical distinctions. With the magnification and sharpened focus of psychoanalytic data there can be movement toward a greater specificity of our definitions and an improved systematization of our concepts.

In general, the psychoanalytic treatment process is more likely, with its magnification, to correct for the tendency of direct observational studies to speculate, to go beyond the sensible limitations of inferential and generalizing formulations and conclusions. On the other hand, the questions raised by direct observational studies will, when they can be studied by the psychoanalytic treatment process, facilitate the theory-building capacities of the psychoanalytic method.

These perspectives have been provided and affirmed by the steady, balanced scientific studies and educational programs of the Hampstead Child-Therapy Course and Clinic. Through the Clinic's deliberate balance of direct and applied psychoanalytic studies, and through its superb mastery of how to organize and reduce psychoanalytic data systematically, major technical problems of conducting psychoanalytic research have been solved. The Hampstead Clinic has the largest, sustained concentration of children in psychoanalytic treatment in the world. The Clinic has originated and demonstrated how to pool child psychoanalytic treatment data and how to classify and reduce the data in a uniform and replicable form. This trailblazing scientific activity has encouraged others to carry out carefully designed psychoanalytic research since these methods have enabled us to compare studies carried out by psychoanalytic investigators in other clinics.

The dissemination of these research activities and findings has been accomplished well through publication and through the highly energetic training programs at the Clinic. Young men and women have been trained as therapists and in research in child psychoanalysis. Many of them have come to the United States and have strengthened our teaching and research programs through their activities as child analysts.

In addition to the large number of children seen in diagnostic and direct psychoanalytic treatment,[1] the following list outlines the balance and versatility at the Hampstead Clinic.

---

[1] ". . . every case accepted for treatment for whatever reason becomes automatically a case also serving research, and the material derived from it is

A. *Direct Observations*
   1. Nursery School for Normal Children
   2. Nursery Group for Blind Children
   3. Well-Baby Clinic
   4. Play Group for Toddlers and Their Mothers
B. *Research* (including the methodological instruments for classifying and reducing the direct psychoanalytic treatment data and their updating through scholarly annual reports)
   1. Profile Study Group
   2. Index of Psychoanalytic Treatment Case Material
   3. Diagnostic Service and Study Group
   4. Concept Study Group
   5. Clinical Study Group
   6. Development of Blind Children
   7. Studies of Adolescents in Psychoanalytic Treatment
   8. Study Group on Borderline and Psychotic States in Children
   9. Psychosis Profile Study Group
   10. Simultaneous Analysis of Parents and Children
C. *Other Applications of Psychoanalytic Theory*
   1. Discussion Group for Nursery School Teachers and Matrons of Residential Nurseries
   2. Discussion Group with Pediatric Consultants
   3. Liaison with the Pediatric Units of General Hospitals
   4. Lectures to Professional Organizations

This simple listing cannot adequately convey the enormously stimulating and productive scientific work of those we collectively call "The Hampstead Child-Therapy Course and Clinic." Many of us not at Hampstead have been able to engage more confidently in direct observational and intervention studies because we knew there were at Hampstead the research instruments, the data base, and the corrective balance to help us avoid the speculative pitfalls of such studies, and to facilitate their useful comparison. In an important sense the work of the Hampstead Clinic has enabled many in other settings to move back and forth between practice and theory, which to my mind

---

used as such systematically, without the two purposes interfering with each other" (Sandler, Novick, and Yorke, 1970).

is the most relevant and productive way of advancing theory
and practice in the understanding of human development and
functioning.

One such important instrument is the Profile which helps us
assess, deal with, and prognosticate more usefully about many
of the new problems we are confronting, e.g., the battered or
abused child syndrome, the children who have a genetic handicap or defect, children with chronic physical illness and children who are the beneficiaries of life-saving cardiac and trans-
plant surgery as well as other advanced medical technologies.
The Profile gives us a replicable, systematic method of making
an inventory of each child's weaknesses and strengths in a
manner that reliably summarizes what we do know and what
we don't know, and of keeping track of the efficacy of the
therapeutic measures undertaken to obtain maximum rehabilitation.

The Clinic's work has fostered collaboration of child
psychoanalysts, pediatricians, nurses, and surgeons in providing preventive psychological care.

In keeping with the tradition of the Hampstead Clinic, to
apply psychoanalytic knowledge when it is needed, I shall
describe the opportunity we had, in a pediatric intensive care
unit, to help and at the same time to study a young child's
recovery from a devastating accident. This report illustrates
how the application of psychoanalytic understanding influenced the care of this child who was severely injured in an
automobile accident.

Chrissy, a 3½-year-old girl, was run down by an automobile
as she darted across the road joyously to greet close friends.
She suffered multiple comminuted fractures of the skull, bifrontal lacerations and contusions of the brain, scalp lacerations, a fracture of the upper extremity, and multiple abrasions
and contusions. This necessitated a wide bifrontal craniectomy,
immediate and repeated transfusions, a tracheotomy, *and
placement in a pediatric intensive care unit.* Chrissy's parents were
professionally familiar with the hospital; as their daughter's life
moved from precarious uncertainty to recovery, one of them
was in the hospital by her side at all times upon the advice and
with the support of a pediatrician and his psychoanalytic col-
laborator.

One cannot speak too highly of the extraordinary scientific and technical knowledge, skill, and competence that literally saved Chrissy's life and made a complete recovery possible. At the same time, an intensive care unit, by virtue of its rigorous monitoring demands, tends to dehumanize the care of patients, especially young children. Psychoanalytic theory suggested that care and recovery would be facilitated by the active participation of the parents. The mortally ill child needed an auxiliary ego constantly available to help her monitor the massive manipulations of her body and to preserve the continuity of the affectionate bonds between her and her parents. The parents also had needs—to help out, to be active in trying to overcome the physical trauma to Chrissy and the psychological trauma to Chrissy and themselves. The presence of the parents elaborated and consolidated the excellence of Chrissy's care by maintaining a close human contact; by facilitating nonverbal communication that enabled Chrissy to know, as she entered the world of the living and full consciousness, that there was a safe and reassuring continuity between the crevice of the sudden disruption of her life and the resumption of it.

What led to a successful physical recovery, in large part, might also have been accompanied by a severe psychological trauma, which our study of this child suggested would have included a severe speech and learning problem. There was a good deal of persuasive evidence (which cannot be presented in detail) that the mother's and father's presence, their availability to counseling by the pediatrician and child psychoanalyst, and their guidance of Chrissy were critical factors in her complete rehabilitation. For example, it appeared that Chrissy's brain damage and her extreme apprehensiveness were involved in her inability to verbalize. It may never be possible, in reconstructing her psychoneurophysiological difficulty, to say how much Chrissy recovered her speech and how much she started to speak after she overcame her fear that speaking would lead to catastrophic consequences. This speculative inference was derived from the observation that she had rushed across the street joyously and was struck by the automobile just as she was greeting her friends warmly. It is not crucial to know how important the cortical brain factors and how important the psychological factors were in this impairment of function. Both were involved and both required attention in the slow, at times arduous, but full recovery of speech. Part of the guiding principles was to assist and support the parents in helping Chrissy to understand what *had happened* and what *was happening*.

Chrissy's mother stated:[2]

> . . . advice and encouragement to us to do all we could to verbalize explanations to Christina—starting long before she fully recovered consciousness—as to what was happening to her, why the bandage, why the cast, why the trache, catheter, etc., and then to explain first simply and soon in quite precise detail the story of the accident, has proved, we think, to be helpful not only in the short but also the long run, i.e., the last two and a half years.

This advice was based on the theory of undoing repressions in overcoming a sudden trauma. It was also based on the assumption that amnesia caused by physical trauma may contribute to the child's feeling of helplessness, an anxiety of major proportion.

> Christina has consistently shown the ability to handle questions from kids and others quite matter-of-factly about why she wears a helmet, has restrictions on activities, and how the accident happened. (She used to tell people, "I have a soft head," which was a little puzzling to people who did not know the technical details!) She never has been afraid of cars, or of crossing the road. I don't know how unusual this adaptation is, but it certainly has been welcome.

As Chrissy became conscious she seemed to understand but was unable or unwilling to speak. Her mother wrote,

> We felt it was somehow related to those few frightening days for her when she was fully conscious but literally could not speak because of the tracheotomy—she tried to make noises a couple of times and looked quite bewildered when nothing came out and then stopped trying; once the trache was

---

[2] This and the following quotations are from letters by Chrissy's mother to the author, and are presented with the parent's permission.

removed, she "decided" in some sense to maintain control
—by rather clearly refusing to try to talk—in this one area,
when she had lost control over so many other areas of
previous autonomy—bladder, bowel, feeding. It was fascinating to us to observe how quickly and efficiently a child learns
to communicate in sign language all of her essential needs.
And it was significant that her first words (after four and a
half weeks without any) were spoken in the middle of the
night when her gestures could not be seen and when she had
to wake me up with "Mama, I want water."

The parents found it necessary to know in greater detail
what guided the professionals in their general precautionary
care and in their planned and deliberate treatment of Chrissy.
Follow-up reveals that Chrissy had repressed most of the unpleasant aspects of her experience by the time she was 8 years
old.

As a result of this collaboration by the parents, we became
more sharply aware of the psychological risks of the intensive
care unit. The pediatric staff became aware that parents could
be helpful, even in such a technologically complex environment, and other parents were selectively allowed to stay with
severely ill children. By the presence of her parents Chrissy was
saved from several well-intentioned errors of care and
treatment—one of them quite dangerous—that are more common than we like to realize in this complex, multiservice
environment of the children's intensive care ward. At various
times Chrissy was under the care of eight to ten doctors and
their nursing and technician colleagues. With Chrissy's re-
siliency and the informed dedication of her parents, it was not
difficult to carry out this adaptation of the pediatric ward.

As Chrissy's mother points out:

We tried to think in more general terms of what were the
essential elements of the experience that made for such a
good psychological recovery for parents and child. It goes
without saying that the fact that we knew full well that
Christina was getting the very best technical medical skills
and care possible was immensely reassuring to us. It is also
true that apart from the first few rocky days, Christina's

progress was always upward and relatively rapid. If there had been any significant setbacks, or if we had had to accept early the certainty of a damaged child, our psychological state would, I am sure, have been very different. We always had realistic grounds for hope, and we greeted each small sign of recovery with joy and relief. . . .

We think we can describe some essential factors in our relationship to the hospital milieu that made much more than a marginal difference to our experience.

1. Our relative ease and comfort with the hospital setting helped us to overcome our initial feelings of extreme bewilderment, fear, and helplessness, which must be commonly experienced by all parents in such situations. This ease enabled us, I think, to do two important things:

a) ask questions, quite aggressively, of everyone. Thankfully we were responded to with openness and honesty on the part of almost everyone. We observed that this kind of good communication certainly did not happen routinely, and this was at least partly because parents were too timid to ask the questions (and possibly the medical personnel felt that if the questions were not asked, the parents must either not have them or not be ready to hear the answers?). The result was that we felt we from the beginning established a relationship of trust and cooperation with the doctors and the staff, which we thought was quite crucial.

b) be as active as we could ourselves in helping with Christina's recovery (which of course was as therapeutic for us as for Christina). We quickly observed, and then acted upon the observation, that we were very much needed both to supplement practical shortages in nursing care, and to provide the psychological elements that only the family could provide. Again we observed that though an occasional family, especially in cases of chronic or repeated illness, acted on these same assumptions, it did not seem to be the case in situations of acute or emergency illness. Either the parents were too stunned to draw these conclusions themselves, or they felt too intimidated to act upon them.

2. As you indicated, the immense specialization and technical expertise involved in medical care these days, especially

acute emergency care, lead to much fragmentation and poor coordination of effort. Possibly most of our worries and confusions could be traced to this situation. At various times, Christina must have been under the care of six to ten doctors from different specialties, each with his own schedule. We managed to survive this aspect of the experience because of a wide network of intrahospital supports (i.e., friends), without which I think we would have been quite lost.

I shall describe how ideally I think such a Child and Family Advocate could function:

1. She or he should plan to be available to the family for several hours a day during the acute phases, including the early evening hours (when other family members can come in). She should use this time to:

2. Keep herself abreast enough of the medical situation (hopefully being present during the contacts of parents and doctors so she can hear what they have been told and the manner of it) so that she can go over the same ground again or supplement where it was not clear.

3. To actively encourage the family to express questions if they are not doing so, and their fears and worries.

4. To actively pursue the doctors herself with questions that occur to her, or that are raised by the parents, of omissions, commissions or confusions.

5. To encourage the family with concrete suggestions to be helpful in small, practical ways and in supporting the child's recovery.

In closing it is appropriate on this occasion to predict that the Hampstead Clinic will continue its scientific leadership in child development and psychoanalysis. As you have shown the way in the past to solve problems in the service of children while advancing our scientific knowledge, we shall look forward to the continuation of this finest expression of scientific and humanistic values in the future.

JOSEPH GOLDSTEIN

The Hampstead Child-Therapy Clinic and Legal Education

The short score of years since Anna Freud and Dorothy Burlingham founded their Hampstead Child-Therapy Clinic brings to the start of the next score a record of achievement —such as has seldom, if ever, been earned by so young an institution. The *score,* to draw on the multiple functions of that word, is remarkable, beautiful, and inspiring. The contributions to the life and well-being of many children and their families are priceless. The contribution to the training of therapists, educators, nursery school teachers, and welfare workers in child development is global in coverage and has an impact which grows exponentially. The contributions to the theory of psychoanalysis, to its technique, and to its method of research are, as Seymour Lustman (1967) has written of Anna Freud's work alone, "difficult to exaggerate" in terms of "substantive importance and seminal force."

This year marks, as well, the 10th anniversary of the Clinic's working relationship with the Law School of Yale University. It is on the impact of the Clinic during this last decade and in the decade ahead, in an area outside its most apparent achievements—legal education and the law—that this essay will focus.

Early in 1962 in a memorandum which I prepared with my colleague, Jay Katz, for the Dean and governing board of Yale

Walton Hale Hamilton Professor of Law, Science and Social Policy, Yale University Law School.

I am pleased to acknowledge the valuable research and editorial assistance of Steven Goldberg, Sonja Goldstein, Amos Shapira, as well as the financial assistance of the Field Foundation.

15

Law School shortly before Dean Rostow's visit to Hampstead to extend an invitation to Anna Freud to join our faculty, we explained why we wished to draw on the learning and research experience of the Hampstead Clinic for our work on the law's relation to the child and family. The memorandum noted:

> [D]ecisions involving the disposition of children in a wide variety of legal and emotional settings present problems which demand an exploration of the relevance of psychoanalytic insights. Such decisions have to be made (or at least are being made) in reference to children involved not only in divorce or separation but also in delinquent parent, adoption, foster care, commitment and other proceedings. . . .
>
> The law has been unable to pour meaningful content into the only guide it has been able to articulate for the disposition of children, i.e., "the best interests of the child." Here where law and psychoanalysis share a value objective, the potential is enormous for meaningfully transmitting psychoanalytic knowledge about the growth and development of children to lawyers, judges and other students of law. Though lawyers and psychoanalysts have long recognized this opportunity, they have not made it real for they have failed to sit down together and work together for sustained periods over common problems. Beyond the transmittal of ideas between these disciplines, we seek to translate these ideas into procedures which at least might reduce the extent of injury to the emotional growth and development of children who become the subject of legal decision. . . .
>
> Since courts and law schools in the United States have become increasingly, though not necessarily discriminatingly receptive, to psychoanalytic studies it becomes important at this formative stage that the law become exposed to the best and [thus] become sufficiently sophisticated to sort out the poor. Only then will costly misunderstanding be avoided and effective communication established to assist the legal profession to understand both the extent and the limit of the contribution which psychoanalysis can make to such inquiries.

What has happened since that invitation was accepted, has been of great importance in legal education and holds promise, not yet nearly so fully realized as we might have hoped, of substantial significance in the design and administration of laws concerned with child placement.

The Clinic has had an impact on legal education throughout the United States. To describe what has happened at the Yale Law School will be to say something about the similar developments which are occurring in different ways and varying degrees at other American law schools—developments which can often be traced to teachers who were formerly our students at Yale and to teachers who have been influenced by or who use for their courses the published works that come in part out of our collaboration.

Numerous visits to New Haven during the last decade by Anna Freud and Dorothy Burlingham have become the occasions for intensive and often exhausting work sessions— preparing teaching materials and conducting classes and seminars in family law. These offerings placed special emphasis on problems of child placement. Initially they were for law students and law teachers only, but shortly became offerings as well for residents in child psychiatry and social workers. Through preparation and the seminars themselves we began to find a common language and to reduce the barrier to understanding which for so long had kept each discipline from intelligently and constructively questioning the other. All of this work, some of which has been incorporated in a book on *The Family and the Law* (Goldstein and Katz, 1965) and much of which has influenced greatly the writings of a number of students of child placement, draws heavily on the experience of the Hampstead Clinic, its case studies, and the psychoanalytic literature of child development. Beyond that, some students of law, including myself, have benefited from the challenging intellectual hospitality of the Clinic and its many opportunities for learning. Probably least recognized, because we have now come to take it for granted, though possibly one of the most significant consequences of the Clinic's presence in New Haven, is the catalytic role it played in bringing the faculties and students of the Law School and Child Study Center together in an ever-developing collaboration—thus reinforcing for us the meaning of university.

Though some of our work has brought us in direct contact with legislators, judges, and members of Bar Association committees concerned with child placement (meetings at which Anna Freud would often creatively tilt the problem of concern a little differently than previously perceived by others with a few words which might have begun, "Based on what we have learned at the Clinic"), there is but little evidence in the United States or in the United Kingdom that much of what we know has been translated into the design, development, and funding of policies, procedures, and programs for assuring that each child's placement be made to serve his best interests, i.e., to maximize his chances of growing up a child who feels wanted.

To dwell on the past decades, except to learn for the future, would be to betray the spirit and life of the Clinic. Thus, this essay turns to the future in order to illustrate the kind of challenge and opportunity embedded in the law's failure to serve consistently a child's developmental needs and to give you a glimpse of a not yet completed volume in which Anna Freud, Albert J. Solnit, and I are trying to develop guides from psychoanalysis for students and practitioners of child placement. We intend to call the volume *Beyond the Best Interests of the Child.*[1] It will provide (1) a basis for critically evaluating individual legal decisions and the varied procedures concerned with determining who is or should be assigned the opportunity and the task of being "parent" to a child, and (2) a theoretical and conceptual framework, not only for identifying and criticizing unsound precedents, but also for understanding and making secure many sound, but frequently unfollowed precedents—many of which were intuitively developed long before psychoanalysis.

To illustrate how this forthcoming volume will address the tension in law about the rights of a child in relation to the rights of competing adult claimants, the remainder of this essay will examine a recent set of English decisions concerning one child who shall be called William whose adoption was being challenged by his biological mother [*Re. W.* (an *infant*) ([1970] 3

---

[1] Published in the United States and England in 1973.

All E.R. 990 & [1971] 2 All E.R. 49)]. The case of William demonstrates, as you will see, not only the extent to which psychoanalytic understanding of child development has entered and sometimes plagued the thinking of judges confronted with determining a child's placement, but also the beauty of the law—its flexibility in construing legal doctrines in transition.

The case begins early in 1968, when an expectant mother arranged with the appropriate local authority for the adoption of her child at birth. As a consequence, the infant William was placed with "temporary" foster parents in March 1968. In September of the same year the foster parents decided that they wished to adopt William. Early in 1969 proceedings for adoption were initiated by the local authority and a hearing was scheduled for April. Meanwhile in March, the biological mother asserted her legal right to withdraw her consent. The Adoption Act authorizes the withdrawal of the required consent at any time prior to an adoption order. The Act allows consent to be dispensed with only if the court is satisfied that the legal—usually biological—parent (a) has abandoned, neglected, or ill-treated the infant, or (b) is withholding consent *unreasonably.* Each of the three courts considering this case affirmed its commitment to abide by the priority of the Adoption Act, which makes the first and paramount consideration in placement through adoption the consent of the biological parent and second and subsidiary consideration the welfare of the child. Yet at the initial hearing in July of 1969 the county court judge, without altering the letter of the statute, was able to change its spirit and reverse the priorities by asking whether consent was being "unreasonably" withheld by the biological mother because of her failure to take into account the child's welfare. He observed:

> [I]nevitably it seems to me that to remove a child from the only home it has known and to put it in care of a stranger would, I think, not only disturb the child emotionally and cause untold tears and unhappiness but there might be a psychological disturbance as well. There is no medical evidence before me but it seems to me that one is entitled to take it into consideration [as pertaining to] the welfare of the

child. [L]ooking at the matter quite dispassionately and saying what should a reasonable mother do in these
circumstances—consent or refuse consent—I take the view
. . . that the reasonable mother should consent in all the
circumstances of this case. . . . I feel she is unreasonably
withholding consent in this case. I order that her consent
should be dispensed with [(1970) 3 All E.R., p. 996].

In May of 1970—two years after William had been "temporarily" placed—the county court judge's order of adoption
was reviewed and reversed unanimously by the Lords Justice of
the Court of Appeals.

[I] cannot escape the conclusion [wrote Lord Justice Russell]
that the judge's decision went entirely on his view as to the
best interests of the child, notwithstanding his self-reminder
that on this point that was not the sole consideration [(1970)
3 All E.R., p. 996].

According to Lord Justice Cross,

The task of the judge in deciding custody cases—and indirectly, therefore, in deciding contested adoption cases—has
undoubtedly been made more difficult than it used to be by
developments in medical thought over the past 20 years or so
[developments, the learned justice might have observed,
influenced, even if only indirectly, by the work of the Hampstead Child-Therapy Clinic which will soon be celebrating
its 20th anniversary]. Before the war it was, I think, generally
assumed that although he might be made temporarily unhappy, a young child would not be lastingly disturbed by
being transferred, even after a prolonged stay, from the care
of foster parents or prospective adopters to his natural
parents if both were approximately equally well-qualified to
look after him. But nowadays specialists agree in saying that
there is some risk of lasting emotional disturbance to any
child who is removed from the care of one woman to that of
another between the ages of six months and 2½ years. They
are not, however, able to estimate the degree of risk nor to
compare that risk with the risk which admittedly exists that a
child who is adopted in infancy may be emotionally disturbed

when he learns later that the adoptive parents are not his real parents. But although the problem has been undoubtedly to some extent complicated by this development of medical opinion, I do not think that the complication affects this case. In the first place as no medical evidence was in fact given, I do not think that one can fairly attribute to the mother the knowledge of Harley Street opinion which she would have had if she had been used to hearing wardship cases. Secondly, even if general evidence not directed to any particular features of the actual case had been given, I do not think that a mother who maintained her wish to retain her status as a mother in fact of such general evidence would be considered to be acting reasonably within the meaning of paragraph 5 of the Act . . . [(1970) 3 All E.R., p. 1006].

Lord Justice Sachs, construing the Adoption Act most narrowly, observed:

To resolve the contests between a parent and proposed adopters on the basis that normally the correct test is to take the course which is in the better general welfare interests of the child is plainly wrong. It ignores the necessity first to establish culpable conduct by the parent. To change to that test from the approach laid down by the Act could entail far-reaching and grievous consequences as against parents unwilling to forfeit their parenthood. It is, of course, . . . open to the legislature after considering those consequences to make such a change. It is not open to the courts, by adopting a 'welfare' approach to the [meaning of "withholding consent unreasonably"] to effect by a side wind a change contrary to the legislature's intentions [(1970) 3 All E.R., p. 1002].

By April 1971 by just such a "side wind" as the Lords Justice would not effect, the House of Lords reinstated the adoption order. With apodictic assurance, Lord Hailsham disposed of the issue:

[I]t is clear that the test is reasonableness and not anything else. It is not culpability. It is not indifference. It is not failure to discharge parental duties. It is reasonableness, and

reasonableness in the context of the totality of the circumstances. But although welfare *per se* is not the test, the fact
that a reasonable parent does pay regard to the welfare of his
child must enter into the question of reasonableness as a
relevant factor. It is relevant in all cases if and to the extent
that a reasonable parent would take it into account. It is
decisive in those cases where a reasonable parent must so
regard it.

* .* *

This means that, in an adoption case, a county court judge
applying the test of reasonableness must be entitled to come
to his own conclusions, on the totality of the facts, and a
revising court should only dispute his decision where it feels
reasonably confident that he has erred in law, or acted
without adequate evidence, or where it feels that his judgment of the witnesses and their demeanour has played so
little part in his reasoning that the revising court is in a
position as good as that of the trial judge to form an opinion.
. . .

[I]t does not follow from the fact that the test is reasonableness that any court is entitled simply to substitute its own
view for that of the parent. In my opinion, it should be
extremely careful to guard against this error. Two reasonable parents can perfectly reasonably come to opposite conclusions on the same set of facts without forfeiting their title
to be regarded as reasonable. The question in any given case
is whether a parental veto comes within the band of possible
reasonable decisions and not whether it is right or mistaken.
Not every reasonable exercise of judgment is right, and not
every mistaken exercise of judgment is unreasonable. There
is a band of decisions within which no court should seek to
replace the individual's judgment with his own.

* * *

Obviously, in a case without medical evidence it is necessary to be extremely careful in assessing any possible danger
to the child from uprooting it from this stable and happy
family atmosphere and plunging it into the uncertainties of
[a new] menage. But, in my opinion, the county court judge
was well-entitled . . . to come to the conclusion which he
reached [(1971) 2 All E.R., pp. 55, 56, 59].

The decision by the House of Lords tends strongly, though not unequivocally, in the direction of making, contrary to statute, the welfare of the child a first and paramount consideration. And, without access at any stage of the proceedings to expert testimony on child development, the county court judge as well as the Lords recognize the importance, as the Clinic's work has so often reaffirmed (Bowlby, 1951; A. Freud, 1965b; Yorke, Davidson, and Isaacs, 1970) of continuity of affection and care to the child's welfare—to the healthy growth and development of his emotional and intellectual resources. And fortunately, in contrast with many similar situations in the United States, for the duration of the proceedings the child's placement with its foster parents—i.e., with the custodial parent at the time the proceedings were initiated—was uninterrupted. William was not transferred, following the appellate decision, to the biological mother only to be shunted back to the adopting parents months later in response to the decision by the House of Lords. He was thus assured continuity—albeit one clouded by the uncertainties of the pending proceedings—of his growing relationship with his foster parents, who by this time, if not when the proceedings began, must be presumed to have become his real, his psychological parents. Thus, even if the Lords ultimately had construed the Adoption Act in accord with the Court of Appeals, its ruling should have application only to future cases. It ought not, after such a substantial lapse of time as actually took place in this case, to exercise, as it would no doubt have, its authority to have the child removed from his psychological parents. Just such a possible consequence highlights the need for developing procedures which protect the right of review while taking into account the heightened significance of time in the life of a child. Final determinations must be made by an expeditious review procedure within a few weeks, particularly when infants are involved, not months or even years as is so often the case.

To turn from procedural to substantive matters, the presumption in law ought always to be, unless evidence to the contrary is introduced, that a child's ongoing custody should be left undisturbed. That means it ought to be presumed in such contested cases as William's, that he is receiving affection and nourishment on a continuing basis from at least one adult (in this case his foster parents); that he feels that he is valued by those who care for him physically; and that he is a child who is wanted, not merely in the sense of want as expressed by competing adults, but additionally in his feeling of being wanted by those with whom he has had a continuing relationship. The burden on a competing claimant, here the biological parent, after so many months have lapsed since the infant's placement with foster parents, must be to overcome that presumption—which is that the adult or adults who currently care for the child are fit to be his parents, i.e., a continuing source of affection, nourishment, and well-being. The other side of that presumption is the presumption that the relinquishing "parent" after such a lapse of time has, from at least the child's psychological vantage point, abandoned him. The burden then ought to be to establish the necessity, in terms of the child's welfare, for altering the ongoing relationship which, if it has not already been formally declared to be an adoption in accord with the statute, ought to be recognized as a *common-law adoption.*

Legislatures, in addition to giving statutory recognition to the "right to be a wanted child," ought to consider establishing guides to child placement (whether the problem of placement arises in divorce, foster care, delinquency, or any other proceeding) a new standard—*"that which is least detrimental among available alternatives for the child"*—as a substitute for the now traditional "that which is in the best interests of the child." Under such a legislative mandate to use "least detrimental" rather than "best interest," courts as well as child care agencies are more likely to confront the detriments inherent in each child placement decision without getting enmeshed in the hope and magic associated with "best" in a way which often misleads decisionmakers into believing that they have greater capacity than they have for doing "good" in what they may decide.

Introducing the idea of "available alternatives" should force into focus from the child's vantage point consideration of the advantages and disadvantages of the actual real options to be measured in terms of that which is least likely to preclude the chances of the child becoming "wanted." The proposed standard is less awesome, more realistic, and thus more amenable to relevant data gathering than "best interest." No magic is to be attributed to the new formulation, but there is in any new set of guiding words an opportunity at least for courts and agencies to reexamine their tasks and thus possibly to force into view factors of low visibility which seem frequently to have resulted in decisions actually in conflict with "the best interests of the child."

At least for the purpose of determining who is parent, statutory guides should force focus by the courts on the impact any extended leave-taking has on the child rather than on the intentions of the adults concerned or their rights. In the absence of specific evidence to the contrary, an infant who has been left in "temporary" care for as many months as had elapsed since William, for example, had had any contact with his biological mother must be presumed in law to have been abandoned for purposes of custody and care. If nothing else, from his vantage point, there had been a critical break in whatever psychological tie had begun to develop between them. Painful as it must be for such well-meaning "parents," their intentions alone were not enough to prevent such psychological abandonment and ought not to be enough to cause the courts to ignore or give less weight to the child's needs which should entitle him to the least detrimental alternative.

It must not matter for purposes of such determinations, why or by whom the implementation of those intentions may have actually been thwarted. Whatever the cause, whoever may feel or be responsible, the psychological fact, which the law must recognize, is that for an infant such as William his biological mother was not his real parent by the time the Lords made their decision.

It is impossible to locate precisely the moment in time when a parent's "temporary" relinquishment of a child to the custody of another becomes abandonment for that child. To put it more affirmatively, and hopefully realistically, it is not possible to determine just when a new parent-child relationship has formed which deserves the recognition and protection of the law. But that new relationship, once developed, should be perceived, not unlike a common-law marriage, as one of *common-law parenthood* or *common-law adoption*. While the process through which a new child-parent status emerges is too complex and subject to too many individual variations for the law to know just when "abandonment" may have occurred, the law can generally verify that the biological tie never matured into an affirmative psychological tie for the child, or that a developing psychological tie has been broken or damaged, and whether a promising new relationship has developed or is being formed. The law ought to presume, barring extraordinary efforts to maintain the continuity of a "temporarily interrupted" relationship, that the younger the child, the shorter the period of relinquishment before a developing psychological tie is broken and a new relationship begins—a relationship which must not be put in jeopardy *if the primary goal of the state is to safeguard the health and well-being of the child.*

Legislatures must, of course, be mindful that a parent (an adult with primary responsibility for the continuous care of a child) may entrust a child to others for short periods of time (with the length of time amenable to extension for older children) and may make arrangements for maintaining the continuity of existing ties without necessarily jeopardizing the child's health and well-being. But there comes a point when temporary arrangements are no longer temporary, when separations are so prolonged that the force of the law must be available to protect, not break, already established or even newly developing parent-child relationships. And such relationships should in law be recognized by a process we would call *common-law adoption.* Such an adoption should carry with it all the legal protections generally available to nurture and secure healthy ties between parent and child.

By thus shifting the focus of decision to the problem of meeting the needs of the child, the intent of the leave-taking adult or of the administrative agency is no longer of relevance. The law moves, as it should, away from making moral judgments about fitness to be a parent; from assigning blame; and from looking at the child and the award or denial of custody as reward or punishment. It becomes unimportant then whether the parent-child relationship grew out of circumstances within or beyond the "control" of an adult claimant.

Though obvious once said, when left unsaid, the limitations of law often go unacknowledged. There is often attributed to the law a magical power, a capacity to do what is far beyond its means. While the law may claim the power to establish relationships, it can, in fact, do little more than acknowledge them and give them recognition. It may be able to destroy human relationships, but it cannot compel them to develop. It has taken the law a long time, for example, to recognize that the power to deny divorce cannot establish a healthy marriage, preclude the parties from separating, or prevent new "married" relationships from maturing. While the impact of a court decision concerning adult-child relationships is not necessarily quite so limited as with adult-adult relationships in divorce proceedings, the court still does not have the capacity to establish meaningful relationships. Here it can destroy or protect such relationships and can facilitate their growth. But it cannot compel them, even though the child, unlike the adult in the denial-of-divorce situation, has less freedom to establish new relationships on his own. The child is far more vulnerable to exploitation by the adult who is recognized in law as parent or custodian. By decreeing that William, for example, be returned to his biological "mother," no court could establish a real relationship between them. Yet such a decision could not be assumed to be a hollow or meaningless one for either of them or for the adopting parents. It would have greater potential for damage and pain for all, than for the health and well-being of any of them.

There will, of course, as in all human situations, be the hard case. But more than likely the law can resolve such cases if it has clarified for itself and the participants the function and purpose of the proceeding and the limitations of the legal process. In so doing, it is less likely to obscure the problem by a mistaken concern for the person whose only special claim to the child rests on a biological tie. Such a tie deserves and receives an initial acknowledgment in law by making it the basis for determining who will first be "parent." But the status of parent, once a child has left "the chemical exchange of the womb for the social exchange" (Erikson, 1950), where law has a role to play, rests on maintaining a continuous nurturing, affectionate, and stimulating relationship essential to the physical and psychological health and development of the child.

Though the status of parent is not easily lost in law, it can exist only so long as it is real in terms of the health and well-being of the child. It is a relationship from birth, whether legitimate or illegitimate, or from adoption, whether statutory or common-law, which requires a continuing interaction between adult and child to survive. It can be broken by the adult parent by "chance"—by the establishment of a new adult-child relationship which we call common-law adoption—or by "choice"—through a more formal legal process we already call adoption. It must be realized that the tie of adoption is no more nor less significant than the biological tie. It is the real tie—the reality of an ongoing relationship—that is crucial and that demands the protection of the state through law.

Finally, it must be observed that these ideas do not constitute a break with the past. Rather, the past is future. There is in law, as psychoanalysis teaches that there is in man, a rich residue which each generation preserves from the past, modifies for the now, and in turn leaves for the future. Law is, after all, a continuous process for meeting society's need for stability by providing authority and precedent and, at the same time, meeting its need for flexibility and change by providing for each authority a counterauthority and for each precedent a counterprecedent.

The living law thus seeks to secure an environment conducive to society's healthy growth and development. That these ideas are not incompatible with legal decisions of the last century will come as no surprise then, either to students of law who constructively resist sharp breaks with the past or to students of child development who have made us understand man's need for continuity.

In language often sounding psychoanalytic, yet written before psychoanalysis and more than 60 years before the founding of the Hampstead Child-Therapy Clinic, is the opinion of Justice Brewer speaking for the Supreme Court of Kansas in 1889 in the child placement case of *Chapsky* v. *Wood* (26 Kan. Reports, pp. 650-58 [2nd ed. annotated, 1889]):

[When a] child has been left for years in the care and custody of others, who have discharged all the obligations of support and care which naturally rest upon the parent, then, whether the courts will enforce the father's right to the custody of the child, will depend mainly upon the question whether such custody will promote the welfare and interest of such child.

* * *

It is an obvious fact, that ties of blood weaken, and ties of companionship strengthen, by lapse of time; and the prosperity and welfare of the child depend on the number and strength of these ties, as well as on the ability to do all which the promptings of these ties compel [my italics].

* * *

Above all things, the paramount consideration is, what will promote the welfare of the child? These, I think, are about all the rules of law applicable to a case of this kind.

The Hampstead Clinic's contribution and total commitment to understanding and promoting the well-being of children is society's assurance that the welfare of future generations of children may be better met.

PART II

3

AGNES BENE

Depressive Phenomena in Childhood: Their Open and Disguised Manifestations in Analytic Treatment

Analytic study of the clinical manifestations of depressive phenomena[1] in childhood points to the many difficulties in the recognition and analysis of feelings and conflicts related to disappointment, loss, and lowered self-esteem. While these affective states frequently appear to be linked with unresolved oedipal conflicts, it often transpires, under closer scrutiny, that feelings of disappointment and loss often stem from prephallic relationships and conflicts, regressively revived by the conflicts of the oedipal relationship. It may be especially difficult to recognize and delineate feelings related to the self, in particular to those of narcissistic pain and vulnerability. A closer examination of these difficulties by a working group at the Clinic repeatedly drew attention to two particular problems. (1) It was noted that in many of the cases studied, affects like shame and painful humiliation were frequently sidestepped in analysis. Often they were analyzed only from the standpoint of structural conflict, and were not always understood in terms of the general narcissistic nature of the disturbance. (2) Aspects of

From the Group for the Study of Technical Problems in Treatment.

[1] Since clinical depression in the adult sense does not occur in young children, and since the term "depressive affect" may not be accurate in all instances, it seems preferable to refer to "depressive phenomena."

aggressive and sadomasochistic behavior were often analyzed from their instinctual and object-related aspects, but not always recognized when they reflected defensive behavior mobilized against painful early feelings about the self.

The analysis of neurotically depressed adults often leads to childhood recollections which may indicate an adaptive way of defense against affective states of disappointment, helplessness, and lowered self-esteem in their early years. These were defenses which did not break down until early adulthood. In the course of treating one young woman, for instance, it was evident that throughout her childhood, her psychic energy was invested in the denial, through ostensibly sublimatory activities, of her lack of a penis. She was the headgirl in her school; the captain of her hockey team; the conductor of the orchestra; and she outdid her elder brother in every respect. In late adolescence she attempted to make love to a woman and finally had to face the reality of her lack, and, in fantasy, her loss. Her defenses broke down and she was hospitalized for severe depression. Similarly, apparently well-functioning childhood defenses were observed in another young woman who entered treatment with complaints of headache and other somatic symptoms of psychological origin. It became evident that her apparently successful, independent, and later promiscuous life was her way of actively mastering an earlier traumatic situation of helplessness. This had occurred when, at 14 months, a very close, exclusive relationship with her mother was suddenly broken when her mother was hospitalized because of meningitis, and withdrew from the child's life. (For many months, during this time of separation, various strange people took care of her.)

As child analysts our cases differ from these adults since something must first be amiss in their childhood to prompt their referral for treatment. Nevertheless, at first sight the depressive features themselves are often obscured; and we have to face the question: in which cases is it essential to work through to early phases and states of development in order to ensure a move toward healthy development, and in which cases will this not be necessary? Our Group was particularly interested in those cases where it was recognized that the child would be endangered in later life, in particular by depressive illness or other narcissistic disturbances, if complex feelings centering around early narcissistic states were not analyzed and remained inaccessible or only partly accessible to analysis.

Before illustrating this with clinical material it may be helpful to outline, briefly, the main theoretical assumptions of the Group concerning the etiology of, and the predispositions to, depression in childhood. There is comparatively little written about childhood depression, though Spitz's classical work on infant's anaclitic depression (1946) and Mahler's important work on the affects of grief and sadness in childhood (1961) are important landmarks. The reason for this is well known. Many analysts doubt whether it is justified to describe the existence of an organized depressive syndrome in childhood, and consider it more correct to see childhood depressive phenomena as examples of a specific mode of affective reaction. This view is held by Joffe and Sandler (1965) on the basis of their study of child patients at this Clinic. I shall not concern myself here with this issue, but I will highlight the main etiological factors of predisposition to depression, the conceptualization of which affects the therapeutic work of our Group.

There appears to be widespread agreement that the basis of depression lies in the first 18 months of life. Its roots lie in a disturbance caused by disruption of the narcissistic unity between infant and mother. Bibring's conceptualization (1953) stressed not so much the oral fixation as the early self-experience of the infantile ego's helplessness and its lack of power to provide the vital narcissistic supplies. The drive element in depression, much emphasized since Freud's (1917) and Abraham's (1916) historical works and further developed by Jacobson (1971) and others, is expressed in the ego-psychological theory of depression, in the importance of narcissistic aspirations and the concept of self-esteem. In attempting to account for the predisposition to depression Jacobson stressed the early disappointments in parental omnipotence, which is often not yet fully differentiated from the omnipotence of the self. This causes what she calls a "primary" childhood depression, a concept first used by Abraham. Mahler (1961) describes how the lack of acceptance and emotional understanding by the mother seems to diminish the child's self-esteem and leads to ambivalence, the turning of aggression against the self, and a feeling of helplessness which occasions depressive affect. Bibring (1953), and later Rubinfine (1962), see the genesis of depressive affect from the point of view of the ego's reaction to an experience of prolonged frustration which elicits exhaustion and feelings of helplessness. This then could be understood as the earliest experience of loss. The experience of helplessness leads to narcissistic disillusionment which disrupts narcissistic unity. It is equally important to observe how in turn it leads to investment of the external environment with aggressive drives. These ideas are of prime relevance when we try to understand and consequently interpret aggressive or what appears to be sadomasochistic behavior. Finally, I would like to mention Kohut's work on narcissistic disturbances (1971). His focus on the development of the self is helpful. It affords a metapsychological framework for the thoughts and experiences discussed frequently in our Group.

Using analytic case material, I shall now highlight briefly certain complexities in recognizing and analyzing depressive phenomena. This is a case of a girl who came into analysis at the age of 9. She was in intensive treatment for four and a half years and in occasional contact for the last seven years, after the termination of her analysis. Apparently Siobhan underwent a marked character change at the age of 5, after the death of her older sister. She had been a boisterous and happy little girl, but she became withdrawn and friendless. Although her intelligence was well above average, she did so badly at school she had to repeat a class. Shortly before her referral for treatment a brother was born to the family. Until then, after the death of her sister, Siobhan had been the only child in an Irish family which had only recently settled in England and which quickly became prosperous.

According to her mother, the early developmental history was uneventful. But, at the age of 3, she and her 5-year-old sister caught what appeared to be a common childhood infection. Siobhan recovered, but the sister remained ill. Complications ensued and eventually the sister died. Soon thereafter the mother became ill with pneumonia and developed a toxic hallucinosis. This was not fully resolved for about four months and she remained in hospital throughout this period. Many periods of ill-health followed. All these incidents date from Siobhan's third year of life. The earlier history is more subtle and difficult to establish, but it is known that the marital relationship was unstable. The father's interests lay elsewhere and he withdrew from the family

One can briefly condense the five years of Siobhan's analytic material into three phases. The first two to three years of analysis were almost totally centered around Siobhan's desperate need to acquire a penis. The next, much shorter period, showed her equally desperate and intense ways of controlling and possessing the analyst and the things around me. The final phase in her analysis, conducted on the couch, involved the memory of feelings of disappointment and despair from the past and the experience of sadness and some degree of resignation in the present. At this time she was over 13 years old. But, from the beginning of treatment, the intensity, persistence, and almost desperate quality of both the phallic and anal material was unusually striking.

In the first phase of the analysis the quality of impetuous urgency, openness, and concreteness of Siobhan's demand for a penis was in the forefront. Her contemptuous denial of the unreality of the demand and the way in which she clung to magical ideas about realizing her hope were remarkable for a girl of her age and intelligence. Her disappointment with the analyst for not giving her what she seemed to want and need so much was taken up with her. Well, yes, she replied; she wondered whether the analyst knew of the magician who put a lady in a large-sized matchbox and before the audience cut the box in half. Finally, the lady emerged with a whole body. Yes, she did think it would be nice if the analyst were a magician and she then asked, anxiously, whether foreign ladies have the same kind of body as the English. She hoped not! How she wished she could have the tall man she saw the other day as her therapist. If she could have him, they could go to a doctor who would give an injection in the man's bottom to make his penis wither off. Once it was off she would take it and swallow it—or would she have to sew it on? On another occasion Siobhan explained that she wanted a "holy" penis, like Jesus's penis. It would look like any man's penis, but it would be especially powerful. Even God would have to do what she wanted, and Jesus wouldn't mind giving his penis to her. Naturally, this material was taken up in relation to her envy of her new-born brother, her wish to get close to her mother through having a penis, and her fantasies of having lost the penis through masturbation. Later, we were able to reconstruct exciting but frightening situations with the father when she had been left alone with him and had access to his penis.

While all these aspects of the analysis were relevant, the central feature of Siobhan's "penis-longing" was not much affected. The degree to which the lost penis represented her lost sister, and her inability to give her up, emerged at a much later stage of the treatment. What aroused the greatest resistance was the analysis of her disappointment in her father for deserting her, in fantasy for other women, and not giving her the attention and care she longed for. This was completely denied. Instead of the resolution of the oedipal conflict, Siobhan retreated into an intensely controlling and apparently sadomasochistic enactment with the analyst. For many months she pursued a game of counting how many boxes she had and how many more she would have to acquire than I had. She counted and hoarded her money, her pencils, and her rubbers. She watched her session time to the nearest second. Her communications were written on bits of paper which she squashed together and then "drip-dropped" into a paper bag. Although attempts were made to interpret the tormenting, controlling, sadomasochistic toilet-training type of situation, and in particular her fear that the analyst would take her precious things and feelings from her, this did little to further the treatment's progress. Evidently complex, unresolved conflicts around loss were regressively revived in the toilet-training situation, along with all the attendant sadistic and masochistic drive activities. She seemed desperately unhappy. In an attempt to help her feel a little more relaxed, I suggested that she try to use the couch, which she did. Initially, it was an exciting and sexualized time for her, but soon a relaxing period followed. It became possible to work through her oedipal feelings of disappointment in her father—but, perhaps more importantly, the all-bad, dangerous, hostile, and hitherto ignored mother entered the analysis. She was finally able to feel some affection and show some understanding of her ill mother. She was also able to see how she had defensively idealized what her father had given her or she hoped he would give her. The early feelings of disappointment in mother were not available in the analysis, since her feeling of need and longing for the mother were not revived. However, one could gradually observe an all-round improvement. Siobhan's school performance reached a good standard. Her interests expanded to include music and sport. She made some friends, though she always remained somewhat aloof. Her looks became more attractive, which I thought reflected an acceptance of herself as an adolescent girl. We agreed to set a date for termination of treatment. In a closing report it was noted that Siobhan tended to react with unhappiness, confused thinking, panic, nail-biting, and withdrawal in situations of stress. Stress, for her, meant a situation of fantasied or real loss. Nevertheless, we trusted that analysis had helped to make progressive development in adolescence possible.

In the seven years following the termination of treatment Siobhan maintained and developed her achievements. She sought me out a few times a year, in decreasing frequency. Usually she gave an external event as the reason for wanting to see me. It became clear that these were occasions when she became anxious as a result of threatened illness, accident, or death in the family. The fear of loss due to her enactments of destructive wishes against herself also became evident; for example, coming to an interview, she left her newly bought shoes in the underground. Gradually, in the course of these follow-up interviews, her attention was called to her enactments in an interpretive way, to which Siobhan responded with understanding. The fact that she does not relinquish contact with the analyst is also significant, as an indication of her unwillingness to initiate or accept loss. Another relevant factor concerns her current relationships. Until now, all her boyfriends were "foreign"; some lived in distant countries and often shared the mother's original nationality. Without the necessary analytic evidence one can only speculate on the extent to which these geographically and emotionally distant relationships with boyfriends indicate that Siobhan is repeating the pattern of her first relationship when she had to be separated and reunited according to external demand.

She came to see me recently. She is now 20 years old. She discussed her boyfriend's forthcoming visit, which she regarded as a favorable opportunity not to be missed, particularly since her parents want her to leave home. This young man might offer her a home instead. There was no sign of emotional involvement or pleasurable anticipation of their reunion. I remarked that I felt rather like an insurance broker with whom she was discussing an advantageous life policy. She knew what I meant and this gave us the opportunity to talk about her anxiety and feeling of unsafety in getting involved with someone in case the relationship should terminate. At the end of the interview she felt relieved and hoped she could allow herself to be more trusting and free with this boy. Finally, I would like to cite a remark she made a few months ago: While her mother sees everything in terms of other people's envy and jealousy, she herself sees the world in terms of people who do not really accept and care for her.

In closing this brief account of the eleven years of contact with Siobhan, it may be useful to examine, with the wisdom of hindsight, certain factors which may have hindered the fuller analysis of the underlying narcissistic disturbance. The failure to work through it is a potential danger despite Siobhan's present good functioning. Her case and her treatment are not in themselves unusual. Because of this some general remarks about factors which might hinder the more complete analysis of depressive phenomena in children may be in order.

There seem to be two major factors which prevented a better understanding of the vicissitudes of Siobhan's earlier relationship with her mother and the disruption of the narcissistic unity with her, which could have formed the basis of later depressive and narcissistic disturbances. I think the first lies in our tradition of seeing analytic material mainly from its object-instinctual and structural angles—a tradition which has limitations. It obscures the need to understand the child from the

point of view of the development of the self—self-experiences
and self-feelings—which could then lead to a reexperience of
the affects of pain and vulnerability. In view of this, one could
perhaps have deepened the understanding of the first long
phase of Siobhan's analysis in the following way. Her impetuous demands for a penis, and the magical omnipotence with
which she thought of acquiring it, could also have been understood as a revival of unfulfilled early omnipotent needs at a
time when the parental omnipotence was not yet fully differentiated from that of the self. One may assume that the
fulfillment of these wishes was originally prematurely interrupted by the mother. Early interpretations of her disappointment in the analyst for not being able to fulfill her wish must
have been experienced by Siobhan as a repetition of the original situation—namely, of a premature disruption of the need
for shared unity and omnipotence with the mother. In retro-
spect, it would seem appropriate to have given her the opportunity to experience this unfulfilled need—not so much with
interpretations, but with the analyst's empathic acceptance of
her primitive wish. The failure to do this may have prompted
the recurrence of premature frustration of her narcissistic
needs.

The next phase of treatment was characterized by
sadomasochistic behavior. Besides understanding her attempts
at control from the standpoint of defense against anal drives,
one can also see how these defenses were mobilized against
early painful feelings. Siobhan's desperate and omnipotent way
of controlling the analyst and the things that belonged to me
came from an earlier phase in her life. This was a phase where
loss was experienced as a threat to herself, since it occurred at a
time when the object was not yet sufficiently differentiated
from the self and thus represented the loss of an idealized
self-object (Kohut's term). Although it was impossible to be
unaware of her despair and the defenses mobilized against it,
the interpretations which were given her brought neither relief
nor increased understanding. Finally, when she started to use
the couch, her crucial feelings of disappointment in her oedipal
father came to the fore. The intensity of these feelings and the
strenuous denial of them indicated that, beside the traumatic

events surrounding her oedipal phase, these feelings must have been reactivated from an earlier time in her life.

The fuller understanding which prevented the analysis of this early phase brings me to the second factor which I think hinders the deeper exploration of narcissistic disturbances in child analysis. This has to do with the analytic situation between child and adult. No analytic process should be understood as an individual event alone. Both the analyst and the child are active partners in the relationship. Hence what the child analyst feels about states of helplessness in children is of primary importance and might well hinder the recognition of the depressive phenomena and the defenses mobilized against them. We know that depression, like anxiety, is a general affect. To analyze defenses against anxiety where the ego actively fights to ward off the threat of disaster is an analytic task familiar to us all. It is often expressed in the child by aggressive behavior which can be trying and exasperating for the analyst. But we feel differently when we attempt to analyze defenses organized to prevent the recognition of depressive affects. Here the child's ego would have to face a state of considerable helplessness, not a threatened but an already materialized situation of disaster—namely, the breakdown of mutuality which the child experienced in the past. This is a painful situation which has to be reexperienced in the transference. Resistance to working this through is great in adult as well as child patients, but there are both realistic and developmental reasons why the working through is even more difficult for the child. The analyst, in this situation, has to walk the therapeutic tightrope of allowing the child sufficient experience of narcissistic pain by consistent interpretation of defenses and allow the development of the primitive search for unity without letting the child fall into the abyss of a paralyzing and depressive state. The situation becomes even more difficult if the child has to face parental rejection as an ongoing factor rather than a historical one. His real dependence on his parents, his restriction in finding a new love object are real limitations.

It is natural, then, that we tend to avoid confronting the child with his painful affective states and instead encourage new identifications and sublimations of aggressive drives. This is why, in cases such as Siobhan's, one can avoid the recognition and analysis of controlling aggressive behavior as a response to early frustration. One often does not recognize it as a sign of "protest" in Bowlby's sense (1960). Perhaps this is what Kohut means by seeing the patient as a *misunderstood,* naughty child, not just as a naughty child. There is a great difference between the two. By encouraging sublimations and identifications we can help to transform naughtiness into something acceptable and good, which is certainly a relief to the child and could even increase his self-esteem. However, where feelings of "I am bad" originate predominantly from narcissistic hurt and frustration, the basic feeling of unacceptability and lowered self-esteem remain unaltered even if successful sublimations take place. It is because of this that it seems essential for both child and analyst to create the opportunity within the treatment relationship to understand the misunderstood, naughty child and not just help him to become an acceptable, good one.

Following this outline of two main factors which appear to hinder the recognition and analysis of narcissistic vulnerability in children, it seems appropriate to mention the difficulty created by the relative immaturity of the child's ego. This is a well-known and much appreciated fact among us, but its omission would perhaps lead to misunderstanding. Studies on mourning by A. Freud (1960), Spitz (1946), Wolfenstein (1966), and others all report a developmental unreadiness in children to give up or to decathect the lost object before adolescence and to accept the painful reality of the finality of the loss. Perhaps there is a similar difficulty, in narcissistic disturbances, in accepting the sudden and traumatic loss of an idealized, omnipotent mother who still belongs to part of the self. In Siobhan's case this early loss was reactivated and obscured by the reality of the loss of her sister and reinforced by the traumatic events surrounding the oedipal period of her life.

Cases like Siobhan, where the disturbance is in the early mother-child relationship, in the disruption of a narcissistic unity which has a decisive effect on later development and is the basis of depressive phenomena, are not unusual. As a result of treatment partial or all-round improvement in the child's functioning occurs. After considering the child's life situation, the analyst is presented with a choice of whether or not to continue treatment. Having considered the degree of severity of the superego functioning and the lessening of the conflict of ambivalence, there are several factors which need to be examined. We should see whether there is any lessening of the child's narcissistic vulnerability expressed in his feelings of shame and humiliation. We should also observe the well-known "playing the fool" and other euphoric modes of behavior which could defend against depressive affects.[2] One should look for evidence of heightened self-esteem or see whether the child reacts with states of helplessness in situations of stress and repeats anew the predominantly pathological aspects of his early relationship—a matter which may be particularly difficult to assess before the onset of adolescence. Finally, it is advisable to examine the child's capacity to bear sadness and to abandon unrealistic aims. If careful scrutiny shows an unsatisfactory state of affairs, the question to be asked is whether sufficient opportunity has been created in the treatment for the analysis of the early infant-mother relationship and the development of self-feelings from the early stages. The child's difficulty in facing pain and his general unwillingness to oppose developmental forces which encourage forward moves are real difficulties, but one still has to ask whether full opportunity has been offered to the child to experience and accept these painful feelings.

I am not suggesting that all narcissistic disturbances can be treated successfully by analysis, or that they are all of a kind and require a similar kind of treatment. Rather, it seems that there are three groups of children with various degrees of narcissistic disturbance. It is important to make this differentiation in order to clarify one's therapeutic aims. In the first group we have those children who are unable to solve their oedipal conflicts and overcome the feelings of disappointment and narcissistic pain brought about by this. By analyzing their regression as a defense against the oedipal disappointment, the child is eventually enabled to face the narcissistic hurt of the situation without undue depletion of his self-esteem. The

---

[2] And which might be prestages of hypomania in later childhood?

analyst usually has the impression that, from the point of view of self-feelings, the analytic task is accomplished. The child is capable of forming significant relationships with peers and is able to cope with situations of stress with some normal altera- tion of progression and regression. These diagnostic points were beautifully described, from a more general point of view, in Anna Freud's book *Normality and Pathology in Childhood* (1965a). She stresses the vital importance of the child's capacity to move forward in progressive steps until he reaches maturity. In this group of cases we usually feel confident that this move will be accomplished (the "ideal" training case).

At the other end of the spectrum is another group of children in whom the narcissistic disturbance is so early and often so continuous that the damage seems to be irreversible. To foster new identifications and open channels for sublima- tions is a justified analytic aim. I have in mind, as an example, an 18-year-old boy who was the firstborn child of deaf and dumb parents, and who is currently in treatment. The narcis- sistic trauma in his case was early and continuous and affected his ego and libidinal functioning deeply. After six years of treatment he can see that his defective functioning is the expression of an unconscious revenge for the psychic injuries he suffered. Although it is essential for this boy to work through his early painful feelings of rejection and misunderstanding, I am skeptical about the extent to which it will be possible to do this in terms of the early states of the self. I find myself encouraged when I see a rise in his self-esteem via ego achievements and new identifications.

Cases like Siobhan's are often thought of as belonging to one of the groups mentioned. The consequence of this for therapy is that either treatment is stopped before the narcissistic pain could be explored more fully, or predominantly interpretive analysis is continued when the narcissistic lesion is deep and basically unchangeable. It is my contention that children who have narcissistic disturbances similar to Siobhan's form a third group. It can be misleading to judge the issue from the child's performance and behavior alone. The adult cases referred to at the beginning are cases in point. They seem to have been well-functioning, successful, and good children. They were able to hide the deep-rooted narcissistic disturbance which eventually came to the fore in adult life with such great intensity. By recognizing a disturbance such as this, and by attempting to understand it from the point of view of the development of the self and from the interaction between the child and analyst, we might, if we treat the problem *in childhood,* reduce the recurrence of narcissistic disturbance and, in particular, of depressive illness in later life.

4

SARA ROSENFELD

Some Reflections Arising from the Treatment of a Traumatized "Borderline" Child

The Study Group for borderline children continues to discuss clinical material provided by the treatment of borderline children.[1] We continue to explore the definition and concept of borderline disturbance; problems in their technical management; disturbances in the formation and function of self and object representations in some of these children, as well as problems of object relationships and affects in such cases.

In spite of superficial similarities between our children, we were impressed by certain fundamental differences in the genesis and structure of their illnesses. Our focus on, and study of, irregularities in the early mother-child relationship suggested to us that some of these disturbances are not necessarily innate, but may result from poor mothering which constitutes an ongoing trauma. This trauma may operate within the mother-child relationship; it may follow on an external event such as separation; or the external event itself may give a further indication of an inadequate mother-child relationship, as was the case in the child I shall describe.

It is helpful to contrast those children who, despite distur-

---

From the Study Group for Borderline Cases.
[1] In the children we have in mind—examples of whom have been discussed elsewhere (Rosenfeld and Sprince, 1963, 1965; Thomas et al., 1966)—we have used the term *borderline* in spite of its wide connotations. We suggest that the term *atypical* is best reserved for deviations from the normal course of development for either internal or external reasons. The term *psychotic* risks confusion with many quite dissimilar disorders in adolescents and adults.

bances in the early mother-child relationship, were able to
develop relatively intact self and object representations with
those children who were either unable to take this step in ego
development, or in whom the establishment of a self was
precarious and liable to regressive merging.

The case to be described emphasizes the distinction between
identification with the aggressor (A. Freud, 1936) and
identification experienced as a loss of self and object boundaries, a merging with the object. Significant events occurred at a
point in the child's development where differentiation between
self and object had been achieved. Ego development had progressed to the level at which the child was capable of perceiving
that the cause of the catastrophe lay in an environmental failure
(Winnicott, 1958). Feelings of sadness, depletion, and anger
arose as a consequence of undue frustration and deprivation.
His ego had developed active defenses which contained an
appeal to the object to take note and attend. In addition,
identification with the conduct of the parents as experienced by
the child became the preferred mode of defense, resulting in
manifestly psychotic and antisocial behavior (Bonnard, 1954).

Past and ongoing reality experiences were of a devastating
nature and contributed to anxieties concerning safety. He
defended himself against these by massive identification with
the aggressor. In addition, the child constructed a "fantasy" of
disaster of a sadomasochistic nature, which he enacted repeatedly and which dominated his total functioning. Analysis
disclosed that this "fantasy," while containing crucial elements
of the traumatic experiences, protected him against a conscious
awareness of the specific source of the pain, namely, the
mother's lack of care and provision of safety.

The "fantasy" also served as a defense against primitive,
oral-sadistic strivings and oral rage; these had been aroused by
continuing deprivations which had been repressed. By lifting
the repression of sucking and biting impulses, their reexperience in the transference helped mobilize the integrating function of the ego. This, in turn, had a favorable influence on his
thought processes and speech which had hitherto been severely
inhibited (Searles, 1969). Thus we discovered that the child
possessed a hidden, secret, and carefully guarded cohesive self.

This boy shares many of the characteristics described in the literature about borderline children, but he differs from some cases in his capacity to establish stable self and object representations. I do not wish to imply that if a borderline child is treatable, he therefore does not belong to this diagnostic group. Rather, I wish to emphasize the diversity of such disturbances. It is my intent to single out a specific group of children within this broader diagnostic category.[2] The work of Schafer on *Aspects of Internalization* (1968) and Mahler (1968) has been most helpful in delineating this child's disturbance. Mahler's conceptualization of the subphases of the separation-individuation process and more specifically those concerned with the rapprochement crisis have clarified my patient's inability to maintain "good" self and object representations in the absence of the external object.

Case Presentation

REFERRAL AND BRIEF DESCRIPTION OF BACKGROUND John J., aged 9, was referred for antisocial, bizarre, impulsive, and unpredictable behavior. He was inarticulate, his vocabulary was limited, and he had a low IQ. Although he was born in England, English was foreign to him since the family was of oriental origin and they conversed in their native tongue. John was the eldest of five children. His next sibling was 5½ years younger.

The parents were middle-class professionals. Both were severely disturbed. The father was schizoid, impulsive, and his needs took precedence over those of other members of the family. The mother, displaced from her own country, felt lonely, desolate, and neglected. She found it difficult to provide conditions of safety for her children and often was out of touch with their emotional and physical needs. Yet her capacity to mother increased as she herself was offered opportunities to be cared for. Characteristically, she engineered violent disputes between John and his father.

Both parents made excessive use of externalization and pro-

---

[2] Dr. S. Fleck drew attention to this point in the discussion and I am grateful for his comment.

jection. When anxious, they tended to react with undue anger which on occasion extended to actual cruelty.

John suffered a number of serious accidents between the ages of 9 months and 7 years. At 9 months, he was scalded by boiling water and retained some visible scars. At 2½ years, he was hit when a car door was opened, his teeth were injured, and extractions were necessary. A number of events coincided to upset him between 5 and 6 years of age. He was faced with the loss of a beloved teacher and his mother who went into hospital to give birth to a brother. Eighteen months later, he was knocked down by a car in the presence of the mother and infant brother.

From about 3 years onward his behavior deteriorated; although he began to attend an ordinary school, he was eventually sent to a small unit for educationally subnormal children. Ongoing analytic work revealed that he was recurrently seduced by his father, who was both a frightening and an exciting person.

It will be clear that the sequence of accidents was not fortuitous but reflected a gross deficiency of those factors which contribute to the "average expectable environment" (Hartmann, 1939), or "the good enough holding environment" (Winnicott, 1958).

DESCRIPTION OF THE CHILD   At the outset, John's appearance showed his unintegrated state. His features were blurred and an all-pervasive id quality was conveyed by means of a heavy, large, and clumsy body and contradictory agility and speed. Tension was discharged bodily in bizarre movements and physical attack. He spat, licked and mouthed all objects, passed wind, and masturbated freely. His clothes were tight and ill fitting, reflecting parental neglect and lack of care as well as the child's own low self-esteem. He could look cunning, calculating, suspicious, full of rage, lost, or withdrawn, vulnerable, appealing, and friendly. At times he could enjoy company and participate in activities. Overriding object hunger was marked, and it was characteristic that anxiety was experienced as an overwhelming threat.

FIRST IMPRESSIONS IN TREATMENT   From the beginning John was acutely aware of the private and special nature of our meetings. He regarded any link with experiences outside the session as an interference and he set a scene for a close and intimate involvement in which the body and the daily care given to it played a central role.

In spite of frequent retreat into autoerotic activities, he was at most times in contact and his behavior was aimed at arousing a response from the object. In this respect, he differed sharply from the children described in our previous publications. Body boundaries were established and the distinction between self and object could be maintained. The need for a caring and safe object was still present and did not have to be revived through treatment (Thomas et al., 1966). He was able to experience the object as one who could potentially satisfy his longings, despite the fact that he was under a compulsion to repeat his infantile experiences and to reenact the frightening, uncaring, and seductive aspects of past and ongoing relationships to the parents.

John's intermittent response to verbalization suggested a capacity to understand simple abstract concepts. It also became clear that he had a capacity for speech, which initially during the sessions had been a mere mumble and whisper. He clearly intended to exclude me and to retain a secret part of himself. I regarded this as a healthy sign, since I knew that he was frequently attacked by his parents without regard to his human dignity.

He eased problems of communication by telling stories. At times, these stories, coming at the end of sessions, had a restitutional quality and were seen as a symbolic representation of an attempt at reinstating a "whole undamaged phallus-body image" (Helen Ross, personal communication). I typed these stories ready for each new session, which gratified and reassured him. Their content remained stereotyped and was concerned with the disaster "fantasy." The theme of the stories indicated John's basic anxieties surrounding the loss of safety and his conviction that he was being punished for offenses committed against the parents.

The setting of the stories varied with events of the moment, from being thrown out into the street to exile in a distant, dry desert where the child succumbed to hunger and thirst. Animals played a part and were usually portrayed paradoxically as dangerously degraded or caring. Thus they represented aspects of self and object representation.

CREATION OF AN AREA OF SAFETY   From the first, I was experienced as a predominantly hostile object. The mere crack in the plaster of the treatment room wall aroused anxiety of panic proportions. He expressed this in aggressive attacks upon me and made a gaping hole in the wall. He also ripped the walls at home, where he was expected to repair the damage with cement which was kept ready for such emergencies. (This ever-ready cement revealed the true expectations of the environment.) I would equate the act of first damaging and then repairing the cavity in the wall with the repetitive theme of the stories in which an offense is succeeded by reparation.

My priority was to create an area of safety within which analytic work could proceed. The approach chosen was based on John's own mode of concrete thinking. We papered over the offending hole. Although he knew that the damage had not been repaired and the damaged wall continued to arouse devastating feelings of depletion, he was nevertheless relieved. The shared concrete activity was accompanied by verbalization of the motivation underlying his aggressive behavior. This was understood in Schafer's (1968) terms as an externalization in the transference of "current experiences with [inner] presences which have originated in the past" (p. 133). Thus we distinguished between the "Tiger-Daddy-John" or the "I-want-everything-at-once-Daddy-John" or the "bashing-killing-Daddy-John." The relative success of this approach was possible only because John still retained the hope that the object would attend to his needs.

It might be argued that the technical maneuver represented a move directly opposed to the classic analytic aim of providing opportunities for the unfolding of the transference. I saw it as a recognition that the transference depends equally on the patient's ego and the attitude of the analyst.

In this case, massive identification had interfered with the ego's ability to distinguish between inner and outer reality and therefore with the capacity to perceive objectively and to appraise the working of the psychic world and of reality. I hoped to widen the scope of the ego, to bring about some delay of drive discharge, and to aid the establishment of an observing function or, following Schafer, that of the "reflective self representation." In this way, John became aware of the need to knock a hole in the wall when anxiety was at a high pitch—a reaction which we came to refer to as a "knocking-a-hole-in-the-wall feeling." The hole-in-the-wall was seen as an externalization of somatically experienced feelings of depletion and emptiness. As the analysis of these feeling states proceeded, his need to damage the wall was reduced to a token action, then to a verbal acknowledgment that the feeling was present, and finally found discharge through verbalization.

In an attempt to defend against the recognition of the mother as an "unsafe" object, "bad" aspects were split off and displaced onto the father and infant brother. In this way we came to understand that the identification with the aggressor (as seen in an enactment of the "tiger in the cage") represented a compromise between his fear of the father's real aggressive attributes and the attempt to deal with conflicts related to his own aggressive impulses and libidinal longings. The choice of the tiger as a representation of the father was most apt. A tiger is threatening, unpredictable, swift, and dangerous; but he is also magnificent, proud, and powerful. One can gaze upon his body at a safe distance, protected by the bars of a zoo cage.

Identification with the grandiose and omnipotent object became part of John's self representation, protecting him against feelings of vulnerability, devaluation, and unworthiness. The identification also served the preservation of the object and guarded against the child's own retaliatory aggressive impulses; it further helped to avoid his perception of the father's disturbance and ultimately of the mother's inability to provide consistent mothering.

John had a gift for condensing his feelings (primary process fashion) into a meaningful communication; thus, he described his disappointment in father who had rejected his reasonable demands for shared interests and activities as: "Daddy's love has run out into the street." The awful feeling that good things cannot be preserved, but run away, compounded his anxiety which was invariably aroused by sensations of body discharge functions such as urinating, defecating, or sneezing. Over-all retention became vital to avoid the dread of depletion.

John's search for a positive response from the object led to his making sexual advances to the father in which John assumed the passive-feminine role. The masochistic aspects of his disaster "fantasy" were acted out and extended onto other male persons in his life as well as onto me in the transference. Here he attempted to provoke a shared sexual experience in which the aim was to be beaten and castrated. My refusal to participate was experienced as a narcissistic blow, followed by loss of contact. He withdrew into a state of sexual excitement and bizarre behavior which clearly represented a turning toward the body in the face of disappointment in the object and an attempt to enact the roles of the two partners of the homosexual act within himself. Interpretation of this material on a negative oedipal level would have provoked further excitement and exhibitionistic tendencies. (This was seen when he contorted his body like a bellydancer.) Rather, I chose to interpret in terms of the body self. For example, his excitement abated when I said that he was trying to show me how clever he was with his body, that his body was a whole body, and that I surely loved him because of that. This example indicates the general line of interpretations which were slanted toward feelings surrounding the self and those concerning lack of safety. Thus we learned that aggressive attack and sexual excitement provided relief from, and were preferable to, feelings of sadness and depression.

The capacity to bear painful affect, for however brief a period, mobilized the integrating function of the ego; he began to talk more spontaneously and the material indicated a move toward oedipal rivalry with the admired, idealized tiger-father. Oral-phallic elements were pronounced and could be seen in the demand for "strength-giving" food so that he could take on father as a rival and an equal. His oedipal sexual fantasies included the idea that the parents consumed vast quantities of "goodies," leaving the children to starve. He described their sexual union as a state of "never-ending summer love," a distortion of the title of a popular song. Once again, John had expressed himself with affect and precision. Exile from this idyllic place was understood to have occurred as a punishment for the desire to penetrate the mother and to acquire her breast-penis. Interpretation of the sadomasochistic intercourse fantasies, which included the idea of the father forcefully acquiring mother's sexual attributes and also beating her, enabled John to talk about actual physical fights between the parents.

The pursuit of positive oedipal wishes was characterized by a growing awareness of the father's disturbance and the dilemma this presented in terms of masculine identifications. John openly talked about his father's shortcomings and his own wish to be different, that is, to please and protect his mother or me in the transference. He longed to be a giant, bigger than the door—to dig enormous tunnels and to perform feats of strength. The capacity to talk of these ambitions was a new achievement in the analysis and represented the first disclosures of his carefully guarded secrets. John also perceived that I was different from his parents; that I was not, for instance, amused by his rather coarse jokes. He searched for a more subtle approach and began to rhyme words such as "sleeper, sweeper, keeper." These words once again contained features of the longed-for relationship and aspects of the self representation. "Sleeper, keeper" referred to oedipal and preoedipal wishes for a sexual and safe relationship, while "sweeper" embodied a reminder of the ever-present anally colored, self feeling of likening himself to a speck of dust that is swept up and discarded.

Oedipal disappointment led to the ascendancy of the identification with the infant at the mother's breast, an identification which had been evident throughout but which now became the central theme of our work. Once again, he found an appropriate, condensed, verbal expression to convey his conflicting feelings, by naming the mother's breasts "Busim" (note the ending "im"). The first syllable is English, the second is the male plural ending of words in Hebrew. Here then was the core of his yearnings—to possess the mother's breasts and the father's penis would mean to be safe from starvation, depletion, and castration. The choice of the English word for breast was significant: indicated a wish for something other than the family could provide and it was a link with the language and reality aspects of the treatment relationship.

For the first time, John became aware of the presence of other patients and he identified with the very young, nonverbal children. Rage and envy of the infant who is permitted to have the "busim" was again defended against by withdrawal into autoerotism and bizarre body movements. It now became clearer that the uncoordinated hand and arm movements had a very specific meaning. Hoffer (1950) suggested that "the hand enlarges the 'mouth-self' to a 'body-self' and thus helps to replace for the infant the missing breasts by its own warm soft body which in increasing intensity conveys the orally rooted sensation of self" (p. 160). It is noteworthy that interpretation of this content was meaningful to John and brought about a reduction of the bizarre behavior and sexual provocation of his father in reality. The overtly homosexual activities thus contained strong elements of prephallic oral strivings.

Immense rage and an overwhelming desire to starve the infant brother came to the fore. He thought of destroying the source of all the good supplies, illustrating this by a fantasy of smashing all the milk bottles in the dairy so that the milk ran out into the street. He cut his hand on a broken bottle and turned to the mother to be comforted and made better. Instead, she spanked him. The expansion of this theme in the transference revealed that John was immensely hurt by his mother's reaction. To be hurt and to be beaten were closely interwoven and he enacted a number of incidents in the session where he repeated this sequence of events. The revival of memories surrounding the earlier accidents indicated that the expectation of being cared for because he was hurt was dismally disappointed by the mother spanking him. For John, this was the *real trauma*. The idealized, all-providing, good representation of the mother had given way to the depriving, spanking, attacking mother, unable to keep her children safe. Recognition of this state was instantly defended against in two ways:

1. By aggression turned against the self. The thought that "all the love runs out into the street" was now understood as a punishment for oral-sadistic, devouring impulses directed to-

ward the mother. To complicate matters, he also identified with the starving infant of his fantasies. This could be seen in the content of the oral intercourse fantasies as well as in the stories he told early in treatment where the offending child is exiled to the desert to starve and perish of thirst.

2. By identification with the mother-cow. I discovered that John spent all his spare time at a dairy farm near his home where he was known as "Jake," the name he had given to the character in his stories. In one of his, by now, rare stories, Jake stole one of the cows. On the way home, Jake and the cow were knocked over and the cow sustained severe injuries requiring hospitalization. The farmer went in search of the thief and was directed to him by Jake's mother, who handed him over for punishment.

The overall conflict is of a positive oedipal nature and the ultimate punishment is castration by the father. It is significant, however, that the fantasy indicated a reversal of the original accidents and an acknowledgment of death wishes directed toward the mother because of the betrayal of her son. Inherent in this story is the idea that the mother cannot protect the boy against the father's rages and that she is, indeed, a party to them. Furthermore, we now understand that the heavy, clumsy walk belonged to the identification with the mother-cow and that the paradoxical speed and agility with which he moved at times could be attributed to the identification with the tiger-father.

The working through of oral-sadistic impulses directed against the mother and the subsequent need to identify with her effected a change in the child's total appearance. Facial features which had been unshaped took on a more definite structure. An onlooker described John as having acquired "a face." This greater integration could also be seen in a general toning down of motor patterns of behavior and a decrease in bizarre body movements. Above all, it could be seen in the manner of dress. Clothes fitted well and were properly adjusted. He took pride in looking smart, neat, and clean, an indication that a change had occurred in his feelings about himself. The alteration in self-esteem and self-regard was accompanied by a greater certainty that expectations would be met and that "good" feelings could be retained and need not "run away." Reality testing improved, he was now able to maintain relationships, and the tendency to act out decreased.

Discussion

In this discussion I shall limit myself to some thoughts on the genesis of John's disturbance and on some problems of technique.

Treatment indicated that the scalding at 9 months was of crucial importance because it aroused unconscious reactions in the mother which further contributed adversely to the already inconsistent pattern of mothering. It seemed that the accident confirmed her own self-feelings of unworthiness and that these feelings were now extended onto John. In addition, her son came to represent aspects of the ill and uncaring husband and his unsympathetic family.

The timing of the next accident is also significant. At 2½ years John had already assumed the role of the father's victim and was often beaten by him.

Brody (1970) writes about the effects that harsh verbal prohibitions of beatings have on the child. The verbal prohibitions do not violate the integrity of the physical intactness of the self; they will eventually be internalized and become part of the superego structure. Aggressive blows, she states, instantly alienate mental processes, offend the child's narcissism in the profoundest sense, provoke counteraggression in a sadomasochistic form, and in due course lead to a need for punishment. It is likely that in John's case the intensity of the deprivations and the threat to life went beyond the limits which could be accommodated by the primitive ego organization. Freud (1924) and Greenacre (1968) suggest that pain and distress in infancy always arouse sexual and aggressive drives—a circumstance that would account for the overwhelming instinctualization which was evident when John began treatment.

Finally, enacting the themes of his intolerable life situation was less painful than facing the reality of having become the victim of parents whom he also loved and depended upon.

It is not clear why John had retained hope that someone would satisfy his needs. One may speculate that the mother-child relationship provided some good experiences, perhaps on the basis of the child being narcissistically cathected by the mother. But we know that John was exposed to inconsistent mothering even before the accident. It would appear, then, that he may have had the capacity to convert a "not quite good enough environment" into a "good enough environment" (Winnicott, 1958). If that is so, it would mean that his ego functions, and especially intelligence, were potentially intact, but had been seriously interfered with by the traumatizations and conflicts.

Throughout our work, I have been puzzled by the fact that although his ego functions were severely damaged, John had retained firmly delineated and cohesive self and object representations. It may be that the degree of energy required to protect the self led to an impoverishment of available energic resources for ego building. A more precise answer can be found in a recent paper by Mahler (1971), which also throws light on the child's inability to maintain "good" object representations in the absence of the object. She suggests that if the intrapsychic separation-individuation process is not allowed ample time to unfold and develop, and if frustrating or even frightening experiences occur in the child's interaction with the mother *after* separation has taken place, "the modulating, negotiating functions of the ego" do not become established, the internalized "object remains an unassimilated foreign body, a 'bad' introject in the intrapsychic emotional economy. In the effort to eject this 'bad' introject, derivatives of the aggressive drive come into play . . . there seems to develop an increased proclivity to identify with, or to confuse, the self representation with the 'bad' introject. If this situation prevails during the rapprochement subphase, then aggression may be unleashed in such a way as to inundate or sweep away the 'good' object and with it the 'good' self representation" (p. 412). This formulation appears to me to fit my patient and may explain the emergence of the first signs of disturbance in the third year of life.

Technically, the transference was throughout the main vehicle of John's analysis. Unremitting interpretation of the hostile introjects once more mobilized the libidinal drives, so that some measure of fusion could occur, permitting the integrating function of the ego to emerge and operate. Furthermore, interpretations were anchored in object relationships, regardless of whether the object was the "self" or the "other," internalized or external, or, indeed, at times a combination of both when he treated himself as both object and subject with the ego once again the master of the drives.

If one regards acting out in life and in analysis as communication and enactment (whether of content, defense, or resistance), interpretation becomes the major tool of the analytic work and parameters can be dispensed with quite soon. Or, as one's skill increases, they may, in some cases, be relinquished altogether.

Summary

It may be helpful to comment on some of the characteristic features of this case:

1. While the child's ego sustained severe damage as a consequence of what he initially experienced as external factors, John's self and object representations were preserved.

2. As a result, boundaries were firmly established, the distinction between internal and external reality had been achieved. Reality testing was basically intact since he perceived correctly that the source of his pain was located in the external world, but secondary interference with reality testing had taken place as a consequence of excessive externalization and projection (Novick and Hurry, 1969).

3. It became clear that marked withdrawal was not of a fixed, permanent nature, but alternated with states of relatedness—John was *still* withdrawing *from* an object. In this respect, he differed from those borderline children whose need for the object was no longer accessible to consciousness. Moreover, he withdrew from the object to the self either in fantasy or autoerotic activities, gaining compensatory pleasure, relief from tension, and feelings of safety. This too is in

marked contrast to other borderline children who have no cohesive self to turn to in states of loss and whose fantasies are often diffuse and proliferate. Autoerotic activities are observed in such borderline children, but we have found that the turning toward the body does not bring about relief of tension (Thomas et al., 1966).

4. One might contrast the motivating factors underlying panic anxiety, which was concerned with the fear of death, with that in other groups of borderline children whose anxiety is motivated by fears of annihilation and disintegration. Here again, the key can be found in the establishment of the self. John had an integrated self, which enabled him to experience the threat specifically in terms of his body and his life.

If one assumes that the interruption of the "circular process" (Sylvester, 1947) has thwarted the development of a cohesive self, then threats emanating from whatever source are experienced both as arising from within and as a loss of part of the self, as "falling to bits." In John's case, the threat was perceived correctly to be located in the external world, although secondarily inner factors contributed.

John had in common with other groups of borderline children the fact that signal anxiety did not perform its proper function. This could be accounted for in the following way:[3]

A. Developmentally: i.e., a signal function of the ego is developed on the basis of enough happy experiences which will build up and contribute to the expectation and hope that its signal will serve the purpose to alert the object to attend to his needs. It can be assumed that signal functions develop only when the relationship centers around well-dosed frustrations and gratifications which are within the child's current capacity to master. Through the resultant internalizations the ego is enabled gradually to bring anxiety experiences under control and to develop its vital function of signal anxiety. Traumatic experiences in early life can interfere with the development of this function.

B. It is well known that the wishes and motives underlying

---

[3] I would like to thank Dr. Robert Evans for his help with the formulation of the following section.

identification are numerous and have been described at length in the literature. Here I am concerned only with two motivations—that of identification with the aggressor and that of merging with the object, a distinction which is not always clear at the diagnostic stage.

I have tried to demonstrate that the key to the understanding of certain borderline disturbances lies in a scrutiny of the child's self and object representations. Clinically, this can be conveyed via the treatment relationship which will differ markedly in the two cases—identification with the aggressor and merging with the object. As has been described, John's initial reaction to me was one of attack, an active move on the part of the ego to ward off anticipated threat. If he had been one of those children whose preferred mode of dealing with anxiety is merging with the object, he would have "become" like me, for instance, by taking over my speech or mannerisms, and this would also have been evident in relation to any person or character who would spark off some anxiety. In John's case, merging was not evident at any point, but he did confuse pronouns at times of anxiety. This pointed to confusion between mental representations or between the roles of victim and aggressor, part of the over-all defense of identification with the aggressor, which is, as Anna Freud has described, a conglomerate of many defenses.

Conclusion

An attempt has been made to discuss the development of a child with borderline features who had been exposed to persistent traumatizations. His analysis disclosed that his self and object representations were intact, but that the internalized object could not be assimilated because it was a "bad" object. It became clear that self and object representations were predominantly cathected with aggression from two sources—on the one hand, from reality, in that he had taken over the mode of functioning of the real object; on the other, from within, in that aggressive impulses were aroused as a result of conflict around ambivalence and feelings stemming from a battered self-esteem. The preservation of hostile object representations became necessary for a variety of reasons, among which could be found the need to control the threatening, unreliable, external object, the wish to participate in the power of the strong object, and the preference for the bad object rather than no object at all.

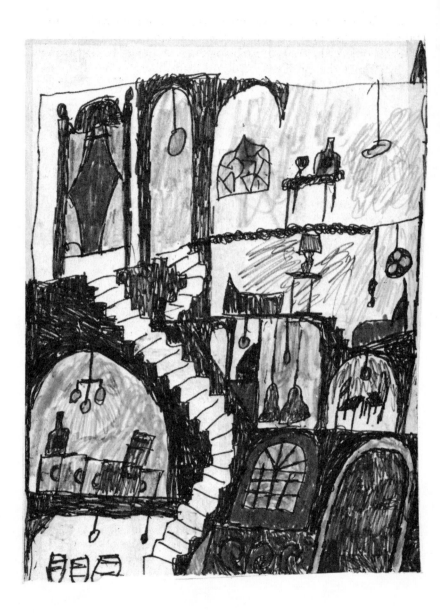

5

MARIA KAWENOKA BERGER

A Threat of Irreparable Damage

This paper deals with certain conflicts concerning the masculine role in a physically handicapped boy. I shall attempt to demonstrate the contribution to these conflicts made by the boy's own handicap, by the impact of his parents' personalities, and by the way in which he perceived his father's severe disability.

Derek is now 11 years old. He is blind in one eye, and his vision in the other is minimal. When he draws, his head is almost on the table, and his field of vision is so narrow that he can only see clearly a fragment of a drawing at any one time. When he is met in the waiting room, he responds to the analyst's voice rather than to any visual recognition.

Thus, Derek finds himself precariously balanced between partial sightedness and blindness. In spite of this, his skill in drawing, his ability to write and read, and a degree of manual dexterity indicate that, even if the dividing line seems narrow, qualitatively the difference between minimal sightedness and total blindness is very great.

Derek's drawings are a proof of this.[1] They could be considered from several viewpoints: as an illustration of his *need* to use his sight to the utmost, i.e., of his way of coping with the threat of blindness; of his *ability* to create beautiful, intricate, colorful drawings; and as a reflection of his *inner preoccupations*. It is on the latter that this paper concentrates.

At one stage of his analysis Derek spent many sessions

From the Clinical Services.

[1] A large selection of Derek's drawings was exhibited during the presentation of the paper. One sample, originally drawn in bright, vivid colors, is reproduced on the facing page.

drawing what he came to call his "dream houses." Their contribution to the understanding of an important aspect of his conflicts over identification proved vital.

The situation from which Derek tried to escape into fantasy was both an external and an internal one. His *external situation* was, above all, that of a child who grew up with a serious eye condition. The firstborn child of a blind father and of a sighted mother, Derek was, at the age of 5 months, found to suffer from optic atrophy. Nevertheless, he retained a considerable amount of sight until he was 8 years old. One day he noticed a shadow in front of one eye, and an operation for a detached retina took place two days later. A few months later, his second eye was similarly affected and operated on.

During the analysis, I witnessed the dread with which he anticipated each of his regular checkups at the Eye Hospital. At one such checkup, at the beginning of the second year of analysis, it was found that he had a cataract in the better eye. Three months later increased intraocular pressure was diagnosed and Derek had yet another operation. His sight deteriorated.

The threat of blindness was a reality from which Derek tried to escape into fantasy, but a problem which he found even more difficult to face was his feeling about his father's blindness. Furthermore, he had to contend with his parents' recent separation following years of marital discord. The parents were of Hungarian extraction and had come to England after the war. Their disagreements often centered on Derek.

It gradually emerged that the mother treated Derek as her confidant and that he had easy access to her bedroom and bed. One also gained the impression that the mother saw in his impending blindness her own denigrated and "castrated" self. One area of conscious conflict for the mother was her hostility toward her son. In the early stages of the analysis attitudes or actions potentially dangerous to Derek's sight were often noted.

Derek's brother, Charles, born when Derek was 3, from the start evoked very different feelings in both parents. His sight, though not good, was much better than Derek's. The mother described how completely wrapped up in him she became. According to her, Derek had been relatively happy until Charles was born; then "everything changed for him."

A few additions to the social history may be helpful. He was born by forceps delivery. He was breast-fed for a few weeks, but, as he was a slow feeder, he was put on a bottle. He thrived, except for a period of colicky pains between 3 to 4 months. Apparently, he took the bottle better from his father than from his mother. He had a bottle last thing at night until he was 4. He started wearing spectacles at 8 months. Nevertheless, he was said to be an active baby and his milestones were normal. Toilet training was not attempted until he was 2. By 3½ he was trained, but his toilet training had been a battleground between him and his mother.

After a brief period in a nursery school where he was unhappy, Derek went to a primary school. He settled better there, except for his dislike of the rough-and-tumble of the playground. He did well at school, but had such difficulty in arithmetic that, when he started treatment at the Clinic, he had no idea of the meaning of numbers.

The parents sought the Clinic's help when Derek was 9, ostensibly because he was staying away from school and needed occupation. He was accepted for observation and the following picture of emotional difficulties emerged: he was intensely jealous of Charles; was unwilling to leave home; had very few friends; was late in going to sleep; had temper tantrums during which he completely lost control; liked to dress up in his mother's clothes, especially her underwear; and always talked about princesses and often dressed up as one.

In the course of his analysis several other signs of disturbance came to light: his many fears (of burglars, murderers, ghosts); his general anxiety-proneness; his tendency to psychosomatic ailments; his learning inhibition—mainly, but not exclusively, of arithmetic.

Intelligence testing established that Derek had a verbal IQ on the Wisc of 133.

Analytic Treatment Material

Derek's internal situation was revealed in the course of his analysis which so far has lasted for two years. Early in treatment, the question of his father's impending departure worried him greatly. Although his mother had told Derek that his father might leave, the departure seemed sudden. The question of *why* his father left had to be tackled realistically as well as analytically. His mother's explanations served only to confuse him.

That Derek's feelings toward his father were highly ambivalent was apparent quite early. For example, he told me that if he knew that daddy had a room, he wouldn't worry; but a little later volunteered: "I saw something on the telly, only I couldn't help laughing . . . about people living in a manhole." The context in which he said this led me to comment on children's anger with their daddies for leaving, on their feeling that it would serve daddy right to live in a manhole, and on their fear that this wish might come true.

At that time Derek also missed his mother greatly. She was working and he worried about her safety. I linked this worry with his own angry wishes toward her. A few days later he said that, once, when he was very cross with mummy, he wished her something nasty, then worried that it might come true. Thus, Derek indicated his fear of the magic power of his aggressive wishes—a fear that proved to be of quite extraordinary intensity. His brother was, of course, another target of his aggressive wishes.

Derek tried to cope with his angry feelings by the massive use of denial. When this was inadequate, he had recourse to reparatory thoughts. He told me, "I like—love daddy the same as if he wasn't blind"—daddy would always be his daddy. "And when he is dead," he added, "I'll leave bunches of flowers on his grave . . . and on mummy's."

The breakup of his family and the intense castration anxiety exacerbated by his eye condition were, at times, manifested through the same wish: that things should be strong "like a rock."

An important reason for his difficulty in being away from mother was Derek's intense curiosity about her private life. He expressed a wish to be able to fly, a wish which he was to state many times during his analysis. He would like to be able to vanish and see what was in other treatment rooms and in cupboards. When I commented on children's difficulties when they are curious about adults' private lives, he said this was not true at his home: if he wanted something, he went quietly into mummy's room.

Before the first Christmas break in treatment Derek told me: "When I think of Christmas, I see a fireplace with an open fire, a clock on the mantelpiece, vases, and many people sitting in front of it in a half circle." My comment that this sounded like a memory was denied at first: they didn't have an open fire. Then he realized that granny used to have one. When I verbalized his wish to enjoy a Christmas, with daddy and granny still there, Derek added, "and Charles." I suggested that the Christmas he had recalled may have been a Christmas before Charles was born. He asked whether babies came to see therapists. The interpretation that he wondered whether I would produce a baby during the holidays led to Derek's asking: "I'd like to know why a baby is bald, without hair." I showed him that this may have been one of his reactions to Charles's arrival and I verbalized his concern about whether mummy would have another baby.

Derek's fear that he might acquire a new sibling was extreme. It showed itself before all Clinic holidays, when his mother was ill, or when she went away. Two main facets of this fear were consistently interpreted: (1) the changes in his life situation and the deep hurt brought about by Charles's birth; and (2) his anger at having no part in mother's love life, and his past disappointment that Charles was not his baby.

Fragments of memories of Charles's babyhood began to emerge: notably, Derek's reaction to Charles's breast-feeding, and his confusion about his brother's sexual identity.

Derek told me that he loved the domes of buildings, and had seen a building which included these the previous summer. It became apparent that, for Derek, this building was a symbol of plenty, of what he had lost. His current envy of Charles, who was spending more time with mother than he, was frequently experienced in terms of the greater number of sweets which Charles was thought to be getting. Eventually, a link was made between the domes of this admired building and those on his mother's body. It transpired that mummy had fed Charles "from the breast" and that Derek had wondered: "Why did she do it?" The fascination with domes in terms of his admiration for his mother's body and a wish to be like her became more apparent as his analysis progressed.

Derek's conflicts over his sexual role could be seen from the beginning. On the one hand, there were his phallic-oedipal wishes, for example, his wish to fly; on the other, there were indications of passive-feminine wishes. In the third month of treatment Derek sought my help in finding a name for his hamster. I said I wondered what the hamster meant to him. Derek replied: "A living creature." I wondered if he was thinking of a human baby. He told me that he rocked the cat and that he wondered what it felt like to rock a baby. I interpreted that a part of him wished to grow into a mummy, and wondered whether he thought that mummy, or daddy, had wanted him to be a girl. Derek's reaction was: "When I was 3, mummy said that in a way it would be nice to have a boy and a girl because when the girl is a teen-ager, she could help her in the house. Only mummy didn't know that I would be helping her."

His mother's unconscious preference was only one of the factors contributing to Derek's bisexual conflicts. His confusion about sex differences was found to be of major importance. It became evident that Charles as a baby was an object of such confusion. In the context of analytic work on Derek's masturbation conflicts and sex games with Charles, Derek said: "Perhaps when we were babies we didn't know what it [the penis] was." I suggested that this "ignorance" referred to the time when Charles was a baby and Derek did not know what "it" was.

Hearing a child in the Clinic hall, Derek passed derogatory remarks about "that girl." My taking up his former idea that Charles was a girl elicited the comment: "If Charles knew what I thought—only he didn't, he didn't have the words. I knew that he was a boy when he started to wear glasses." Derek did when he was out of nappies. I commented on how much Derek must have minded that Charles did not wear glasses as a baby; that he did not have to undergo operations later on. Derek tried to deny this, saying Charles, too, was short-sighted.

The fact that his mother was the only person with good sight in his family caused Derek to see her as endowed with phallic attributes. In a dream, some aspects of which were interpreted in the transference, she was half-Japanese, "a cat-girl." She had fur on her legs and head, a flower in her hair, and wore a red bathing suit. Her husband had a moustache and was very big and fat. He too had fur, the flower on his head was sloping down, his suit was bursting, and his slippers were split. She was against the human race. "There was me and Mike and Vicky [Derek's friends] and she was jealous of our skin. She kept ordering us about, told us to peel potatoes—we had to do things for our keep." The dream contained Derek's images of both parents: the "cat-girl" mother and the big, but castrated, father. At this stage of the analysis only feelings about his mother were interpreted, e.g., that she was jealous of his penis and that she had a hidden one.

Derek's complex feelings toward his mother—his sexual wishes toward her, his envy of and anger with her, his difficulty in being away from her, and his great dependence on her —were expressed in the material from the beginning of his analysis, much of it in the transference. Oedipal wishes toward the mother were poorly defended. Derek could not understand why big sons could not marry their mothers. "What if they did and people didn't know?" he said, "Mummy might want to."

However much he wanted to marry his mother, Derek became aware of also wanting to marry his father. When he vented his fear of burglars, and I said that children sometimes wanted to steal something, Derek replied: "Daddy, so I could marry da . . . I mean mummy." Similarly, his wish to possess his mother totally conflicted with his wish for a new one. When I had a cold, he wondered whether he would see another therapist if I was taken ill. He was afraid I might leave suddenly. On this occasion I took up his fear that his mother might leave. "She won't," he replied, "I asked her" and, he added, "if she did, she would make sure we were in good care."

His family romance came into the open. "I'd like to be with Charles where there is a mother and father," Derek said. Later material often reflected wishes to live with one or another family he knew.

During the fourth month of the analysis I was absent for a few days, following which Derek had tonsillitis with high temperature and deliriousness. On his return, he revealed: "When I was ill and looked out of the window for a long time, it grew bigger and bigger. When I was 6, I saw a cake growing bigger and bigger, it wanted to eat me." Right now things still looked big and he had to look away. He wished they would "go down . . . or up." I linked this with his erections, with seeing daddy's penis, with his wish to steal it, and with his fear that daddy would take Derek's. When I then took up his reaction to seeing mummy's big body, he said: "I know when her body was big, when she was pregnant." I commented that he felt she had eaten a big cake and he wanted it too. The interpretation of his conflict over his wish to grow into a man with a big penis on the one hand, or into a woman with a baby on the other, was met with a statement of resignation: "I have to make the best of what I am."

A new theme now appeared in his material, namely, his thoughts about the part which his father had played in bringing about his eye condition. During the fifth month of analysis, a postoperative repair had to be carried out, and this was done painlessly at an outpatient facility. But before he was taken there, Derek's fear of blindness was intense. He described how they had played catch at school. In this game he was the father who chased babies. We established that daddy used to chase him and Charles. When I concluded that he was afraid of daddy's punishment, Derek wondered why: "Because I wanted to tear off his wee-wee-maker?" He thought it was sad that daddy could not see. I agreed with him that it was difficult to have a blind daddy and I took up his feeling that his eye trouble was a punishment by daddy, that daddy wanted him to be blind.

A wish to be blind came to the fore. As Derek put it, he would then know something (Braille) which mummy knew only a bit and Charles not at all. Also, he wished to compete with his father: So I can take his place." Only very rarely, at this stage, did Derek's other image of his father, as a helpless person, come to the fore, and when it did, it was highly defended. For instance, he once said: "He eats like an ordinary, sighted person . . . except when he has a mouthful of nothing."

After seeing his favorite building with domes, Derek spent several sessions drawing it. He made sure that he drew poles on top of the domes. He talked about the picture of this building on television, which, he thought, was wrong, because it did not have such poles. My interpretation dealt with his feeling that I had been wrong in telling him that women had no penises. I also pointed to his wish to have both breasts and a penis.

After Charles's birthday party Derek drew a house in which he would like to live. It had only one bed in the children's room and the kitchen was full of food cupboards. Later, he drew houses industriously, and this became his main occupation for many weeks.

An important theme which was worked on during the intervening months was that of his masochism and its link with his wish to be blind. Although this wish was also connected with Derek's identification with the oedipal father, as the analysis progressed one could see that, additionally, it was linked with his wish to be "castrated." Before a particularly worrying checkup at the Eye Hospital Derek, afraid of yet another operation, said: "I suppose I'll have many operations, tonsils, appendix." When I interpreted his fear that his penis might be taken out, linking it with his expectation of punishment, he asked: "You mean I want to?" In the same session he finished a story which he had started at school. It was about two girls and a boy entering a spooky palace. He wrote that a girl had tripped up. When I took up the subject of tripping, Derek became resistant. I told him I had learned from his mother that he had slipped on some steps during a walk and had been angry with her. "It's so embarrassing," he responded, "I know you'll say that I want to pretend I can see." I said I had told his mother he was right in being angry, because she had not warned him about the steps.

His wish to slip became apparent. Summer holidays were approaching and Derek was to spend a week with family friends. He worried that something might happen to his eyes. I connected his wish to get blind with a wish to be hurt and with a wish, expressed in a dream, to be magically changed into a girl. "I want my eyes to be hurt?" he asked. His understanding was clearly shown when, in response to my question about what I should wish him for the holidays, he said: "Not to slip because of those thoughts."

At this point one might raise the question why, in a boy whose mother considered him to be more powerful than his father, a wish to be hurt and blind should be connected with a feminine wish. Perhaps the answer is to be sought in the fact that Derek's identification with his mother included both her phallic and "hurt" aspects. Thus, to be blind and hurt may have meant to Derek to possess the "castrated" features of his father as well as the "hurt" aspects of his mother. In addition, there was his need for punishment. But the matter was further complicated by his identification with the powerful oedipal father, one of whose attributes was that *he* was *blind*.

Toward the end of the first year of analysis Charles was suddenly taken to hospital. It was nothing serious, but when Derek came home, his mother and Charles were not there. The subsequent analytic material reflected the revival of memories of mother's hospitalization for Charles's birth.

During this week of Charles's illness Derek started to draw houses again. The first of these drawings showed Charles's room under a dome, while Derek's room was connected with every part of the building by lantern-lit passages and staircases. There was no bedroom for his mother, but there were several dining and sitting rooms and a well-equipped kitchen. Derek called this drawing "A rich man's house." Indeed, all his houses were characterized by their opulence. When he drew his next "dream house," I commented that he was running away from the house he *did* have. In this version of the house there were several servants' rooms. The servants, Derek explained, would make his bed, put him to bed. As he was wearing a latch key on a string that day, I verbalized his wish for somebody to be always there, to care for him, feed him, and cuddle him. He responded with an attempt at denial: mummy still cuddled him. He commented on the many staircases he had drawn, and we established links with his godmother's posh house.

The wish expressed by the "dream houses" was consistently interpreted as a return to his "paradise lost," to the time before Charles was born and Derek could still see well. There was, however, an important element of this "paradise" which was not yet understood. It concerned Derek's feelings about his father. At one level we knew that he wanted his father back, but we also knew that he could not accept his feeling that his father was unsatisfactory. Derek's longing for his father had a strong negative-oedipal component.

From the many staircases in his houses, a symbol of richness, sometimes referred to as "gigantic," we could understand Derek's questions about his father's masculinity: about "baby seeds." They also provided a clue to understanding his concern about erections and masturbation, including anal masturbation.

A few weeks after the discovery of the cataract, as Derek was drawing yet another dream house, it was possible to reconstruct the impact which his father's blindness had on Derek. He recalled playing on the stairs of his godmother's house. This led to the understanding of his fear of stairs, for example, of the Clinic front steps. Derek stated: "If I had two wishes, I'd wish not that I should see better, but that daddy should see." When I asked what daddy was like on stairs, Derek's reply was: "Oh, he is very good, he is used to them." "And in the old house?" I asked (the family had moved when Derek was 3). He replied that it had no stairs, and volunteered: "I remember my bedroom when we moved to this house. I slowly climbed up the stairs, the bedroom was empty, had no furniture, it was sort of mauve." I said that, perhaps, it was the first time that he had noticed that his daddy climbed stairs differently from other daddies and realized that he was blind. "He wasn't used to it yet," Derek thought. I added that the experience might have made him feel empty inside, deprived him of the idea that daddy could see. Derek said he wished he had not done something he used to do, i.e., run when daddy would want to take him on his knees. I could show him his old fear of daddy's blindness.

The subject of "daddy on the stairs" became a central one in his analysis. It came to symbolize Derek's image of his father as helpless. The material which came straight after the reconstruction revealed Derek's anger with the blind father. He drew a staircase in which each step was of a different color. I compared it with his grin—a constantly used defense against feelings of sadness or anger—and reminded him that he might have been afraid when he saw daddy groping his way on the stairs. He claimed he did not remember anything about it. The verbalization of his fear of blindness was met with a quotation from his mother that he would see better after the cataract operation. I approached the issue in terms of "we hope," and Derek asked me to tell his mother not to talk the way she had done. He drew a "royal staircase," saying, "Daddy groped his way, he could fall." When I took up his former wish to push daddy down the stairs, he replied with feeling: "If he does not come to see us soon, I would feel like doing it."

A few weeks later the diagnosis of raised intraocular pressure was made. The period before the operation produced a lot of material connected with blindness in general, and father's blindness in particular. Derek's guilt feelings about his aggressive wishes toward his father were intense. The staircases he constantly drew now represented his fear of falling down as well as his wish to do so and be blind like father. In this wish we saw an identification with the "castrated" as well as with the manly aspects of father. Derek drew a two-headed monster and recalled that his friends used to ask him why his daddy's eyes were open, if he was blind. And yet, Derek saw his wish to fall down the stairs and be blind as: "To be like daddy, be a man."

He asked his mother point blank if he would be blind when he grew up and she answered that he would. He saw the forthcoming operation as a punishment for his aggressive wishes. He asked me what I thought of his father. Derek's own thoughts were expressed thus: "I sometimes love him terribly; sometimes I hate him terribly, and sometimes I love and hate him."

When the time of the operation came Derek coped with it very well. Unfortunately, he now saw less well than he used to. Nevertheless, when he saw me off after I had visited him in the hospital, he ran down a flight of stairs with great speed. He explained that he had counted the steps.

Derek tried hard to do things he used to do, e.g., draw. Among his current worries there was one about eating: "It isn't easy to eat if you don't see well." When I took up his concern that he would eat like daddy, he was reminded of what I had said about daddy groping his way on the stairs.

He increasingly voiced his fears about his future, saying, for example: "Sometimes I think I'll marry and have a wife and children; sometimes that I'll have a wife and no children; sometimes, that I'll have children and no wife; and sometimes that I'll be a bachelor, with a dog." I thought he wanted to be both a mother and a father, and he agreed with me.

During a period of the analysis when we were working through Derek's fears of his aggression and of growing up, he related a fantasy concerning a house near the Clinic which he liked. In this fantasy he was a grown-up man, then became a teenager, then a boy who currently lived in this house. "Growing down, instead of up," as he put it. When we discussed his wish to be a baby, he expressed fears of being alone when his parents died; of adult marital relationships which end up in divorce; and of dying. A dream reflecting his death wishes against his parents and against Charles indicated the essential reason for his preoccupation with death.

One could now see the part which Derek's fear of his father played in his inhibition of aggression and competitive strivings: a fear connected with his father's blindness and impulsiveness as well as with Derek's projection of his own aggressive-castrating wishes onto the father.

He feared the start of the new school year "because they all play games." While playing draughts with me he remarked on my "sly plans." The verbalization of his fear that an opponent might harm him elicited the reply that this could happen "if we were draughts, if these were armies." When I took up the projection, Derek stated: "There is violence in me." I agreed that there was, in his wishes. It emerged that Derek wanted to appropriate "daddy's things." I could then show him how he displaced onto other boys his fear of his father, which stemmed from his wish to take father's penis away from him.

The acquisition of a new toy, a rather special "click-clack," appeared to initiate some change in this area. Derek became an object of his classmates' envy. However, he in turn was envious of their skill with this toy. When he first demonstrated it to me, he described how good other boys were at reversing it, which he could not do. He complained that the noise was like that of a machine gun. After his fear of being "machine-gunned" or of "machine-gunning" others was taken up, he could reverse the toy without difficulty.

Soon afterward he decided to go swimming in the pool used by the school. He did not go with his classmates, but went with another boy and the boy's special teacher. This was the first time he had used the school's pool. He proved to be a good swimmer.

The released and sublimated phallic exhibitionism began to find more emphatic expression. Derek's drawings, his collection of books on architecture, have earned him his teachers' and schoolmates' admiration.

Summary and Conclusions

An attempt has been made to describe conflicts over identification in a boy whose development from infancy onward was affected by his poor sight; by a life with a father who was both blind and highly ambivalent toward the child; by life with a mother for whom a "defective" son was an offense; and by life with a better-sighted brother who was highly valued by both parents.

The sequence of events between the ages of 3 and 3½ appears to have been especially pathogenic: the move to the new house, the ensuing full realization of the father's blindness, and Charles's birth a few months later. It would seem that Derek had retreated from a tenuous positive-oedipal phase to an anal fixation point. Phallic-exhibitionistic and competitive and aggressive wishes became grossly inhibited. Fears of his blind father and of his mother's rejection of his masculinity played a large part in this. Defensively, Derek identified with his mother, his "lost" love object. The operations and the diminished sight may have pulled him still closer to a passive-feminine, masochistic solution. On the other hand, his parents' separation, coupled with mother's seductiveness, made fantasies of sexual partnership with her ostensibly realizable. In the new family situation Derek's fantasies seemed to oscillate between wishes to be his mother's husband, her daughter, and father's female partner.

Although there is still a considerable amount of work to be done on his fears of masculinity and aggression, Derek has become a much more lively boy and much less of his mother's shadow. One now sees in the transference the revival of intense wishes to compete with his father as well as the sadomasochistic quality of his relationship with his mother.

Derek's use of denial of affect and reality which, together with reversal of affect, used to be his major defense, has diminished considerably. When Derek talks about the threat of blindness, he shows anger, envy, fear. He insists on saying *"when* I am blind," rather than *"if,"* ostensibly in order not to have false hopes. One could ask whether, in the case of a child threatened with blindness, it was right to analyze his defense of denial. My answer would be that for some partially sighted children, it may not be right, but for Derek it seemed proper. His ability to talk about blindness with me and with his mother appears to have made him somewhat more emotionally prepared for it, while the undoing of the denials surrounding his father's blindness enabled him to understand that there were some objective reasons for his fear of, and anger with, his father. One practical outcome of the decreased use of denial is that Derek has become better able to ask for help in situations which he cannot manage alone.

There is a narcissistically depleted core in Derek, manifested in his extremely low self-esteem, in gestures of self-cuddling when he feels lonely, and in his regressive wishes. These wishes, often expressed in oral terms, could be understood as rooted either in an unsatisfactory early feeding situation or in envy of Charles's early feeding. I am inclined to the latter view.

What must have affected his well-being in the first year of life was his parents' reaction to the discovery of his eye defect at 5 months. Their decathexis of him after Charles's birth and the deterioration of his sight later on dealt severe blows to his self-esteem, which was already precariously balanced.

When Derek feels depressed about his future, one finds it difficult to find things in it to which he can look forward. Perhaps his rich fantasy life, which in the past perpetuated a belief in the omnipotence of his wishes and facilitated denial in fantasy, will be an aid to him. In a fantasy which he recently described, Derek had lost his sight at 17, was married, and was the organizer of a permanent exhibition of architectural pictures. The pictures were "gigantic" and were kept in "gigantic" cases. His wife was very nice, and not like anyone he knew.

6

CLIFFORD YORKE, RENATE PUTZEL,
and LORE SCHACHT

Some Problems of Diagnosis in Children Presenting with Obsessional Symptomatology

In the last few years we have become particularly interested in the intricate relationship between the surface manifestation of symptoms and the underlying pathogenic processes and influences. This interest has been further stimulated by Anna Freud's recent paper on "Symptomatology in Childhood" (1970).

Recently, a number of children suffering from obsessional symptoms have been referred to us for assessment. None of them, however, has turned out to have a typical obsessional neurosis. In this paper we shall refer to five such cases, though more detailed clinical illustration will be confined to two of them. We hope they will indicate the variety of underlying pathology to be found in such cases. In addition, we shall try to suggest how they differ from the more typical obsessional neuroses in childhood.

In what follows, it will be useful to bear in mind the characteristic features of obsessional neuroses as they have been

From the Group for the Study of Diagnostic Assessment. The discussions which went into the preparation of this paper took place among the members of this group, and the cases chosen as clinical illustrations had undergone diagnostic assessment by them. In this sense, then, the real authorship of the paper belongs to the group, while the writers have translated some of the group's thinking into a formal paper.

classically described—in recent times by Anna Freud (1965a, 1966). When this relatively clear and familiar structure is compared with our present cases, important deviations will be found.

Typical Features of Our Cases

In contrast with this classical childhood neurosis which often develops insidiously, there was, in all our cases, an acute onset of pronounced obsessional symptoms which led to urgent referral. The family was unable to tolerate the child's behavior. This was partly due to the unfamiliar character of the symptoms, so unexpected by the parents; a large measure of urgency stemmed from the sudden emergence of the child's demanding and controlling behavior, generally experienced by the family as an aggressive attack. Closer examination, however, showed that the child's motivation was not necessarily aggressive.

It was also striking that, in three of our cases, some of the most disturbing symptoms disappeared as quickly and unexpectedly as they had begun, even though such symptoms gave way to others. It is also of interest that none of our patients had an obsessional character structure. The average age of our patients at the time of acute onset was between 9 and 13. All of them were either approaching, or had just reached, puberty, with the exception of a somewhat backward girl of 16.

There is another point we want to make: in the classical obsessional neurosis we expect a high degree *of symbolization and intellectualization,* with the disturbance located in the thought processes themselves. This is commonly associated with the high intelligence and precocious ego development found in the obsessional neurotic. None of our children showed particularly good intelligence: their verbal IQ's ranged from 80 to 120. A pronounced step from body to mind, in the sense of mentalization, was not a characteristic feature of their disturbance.

On the other hand, the preoccupation with *real dirt* and feces was intense. We sought to understand the extent to which the child tried to defend against *dirt itself, thoughts of dirt,* or some specific *meaning* of dirt. All these children avoided dirt in a very concrete sense, though for widely differing reasons. In four of our five cases *compulsive hand-washing* was a leading symptom. In the one case where this symptom was missing, a specific religious rule, namely, the placing of water by the bedside for washing, may have made such a symptom unnecessary.

The marked involvement of the external world in the disturbance also caught our attention. While the true obsessional neurotic has gained a certain measure of independence of the object world, and may try to hide his suffering with varying success, the opposite was true of our patients.

There were doubts whether, in these children, ego and superego reached a sufficient degree of maturity to enable them to tolerate and find appropriate drive expression. Certainly, their superego development had not reached the high level of structure and independence expected in the typical obsessional neurotic; and their objects were used for both ego and superego support in their inner struggles. We have chosen for our clinical illustrations the two most contrasting of our five cases—one child whose clinical picture comes nearest to that of an obsessional neurosis and yet is far from identical with it, and another whose underlying pathology is furthest removed from the more typical disorder. The first, Ron, was 13½ at the time of diagnostic assessment and he was subsequently taken into analysis. The other child, Amy, was 16 when her symptoms began and was taken into psychotherapy when she was referred to us two years later.

CASE 1 Ron was referred to this Clinic with severe obsessional symptoms. Tall for his age, he was blue-eyed and rather pale. He showed occasional glimpses of a humorous impishness during interview. In talking to the psychiatrist, he would underline his words with expressive movements of his right hand. Indeed, he became quite lively; at one point he took his cap in his left hand and made it dance on his outstretched forefinger, looking at the doctor and smiling in a friendly manner.

The onset of Ron's symptoms was sudden. Immediately after his Bar Mitzvah, he was ill for a week with gastric flu. While in bed he occupied himself with books on the Jewish law. He became so absorbed in ritual prayers that he had no time to eat, to talk to his mother, or indeed to do anything else. If he made a mistake in his Hebrew, he started the day's prayers all over again. His refusal to eat resulted in considerable loss of weight. At his grandparents' suggestion the mother and Ron talked to the rabbi. This helped a little and his prayers began to decrease, to be gradually replaced by a preoccupation with dirt. He became terrified that dirt from under his fingernails or his saliva would drop on the floor; and that, by making the floor slippery, others would fall and injure themselves. Before going to school, and before even leaving the room, his mother had to make sure there were no bits of food, dog's excrement, or other dirt sticking to his shoes.

Shortly after he was told in a *Schiur*—a lesson in religious knowledge—not to touch women, he carried the interdiction to such lengths that he refused to queue for lunch in case he had to stand next to a girl. He avoided crossing roads, fearing that he might fail to notice a car and so be run over. On his way to school Ron phoned his mother at regular intervals, and again when he got to school, to make sure she was still alright and had not fallen on anything he might have dropped.

Ron was an only child. He was conceived during a brief reconciliation in an unhappy marriage, after the mother had threatened to leave the father because the latter's refusal to work had led to crippling financial problems. His birth apparently initiated a complete deterioration in the parents' relationship; they finally separated when Ron was 4½.

After the separation, there were in fact episodes of encopresis. At this time, Ron lived with his mother in a residential Jewish college where she worked as a nurse, and he was often left to his own devices. His mother found feces hidden behind curtains and under rugs. His increasingly disturbed behavior soon made it impossible for Ron to stay. He was now sent to a children's home where he stayed for the next four years. The mother said that in many ways this new situation was easier for Ron. He seemed happier and far more relaxed; but she saw little of him, particularly during the first six months, and her view must be treated with caution. When she took Ron at 11 years to live with her, she felt again that perhaps she and Ron were "not good for one another," but she regarded it her duty to stay with him.

At 10, while still in care, Ron was hospitalized twice because of an operation for an undescended testicle. At 12 he was again in the hospital for a dental operation.

We now come to an episode we think very significant. Ron had suggested inviting his father to his Bar Mitzvah. While waiting for his father to ring him, he found a note from his mother instructing him to tell his father he could not invite him. Ron was extremely upset, but did as his mother ordered. When she returned home she found he had wet his trousers. Until his analysis began, these matters were never mentioned by mother or son. The Bar Mitzvah passed uneventfully, but immediately afterward his symptoms began. At this time Ron became interested in orthodox Jewish religion, and spent most of his evenings learning Hebrew and studying the Torah. We shall shortly consider, in comparing our two cases, Ron's preoccupation with law in relation to the functioning of his superego.

Ron, who had been told that his father was on holiday when his parents finally separated, learned "gradually" that he would not be coming home again. It seems likely that Ron came to believe that his oedipal death wishes toward the father had indeed killed him. The coincidence of the father's departure and Ron's oedipal phase must have aroused grave anxiety, and a resulting regression was seen in the encopresis. The reemergence of these conflicts in puberty, when his father was once more banished, this time from the Bar Mitzvah, played a precipitating role in symptom formation. The father was now idealized as the awaited Messiah, who will forgive him and put an end to all wars.

In response to the TAT cards, Ron told two stories which obviously relate to these conflicts and which are both interesting and revealing:

[Boy leaning on bed with head on arm]
Henry was reflecting on what he had done. He was sorry about it and realized that this would change his whole life.

He would like to have thought as if nothing had happened. He had to face the grim reality of what he had done and how it would affect him. He didn't really care about how it affected others, although he was very concerned about the way his life would change. He was sorry he did it, he had only meant it as a bluff to get some money out of the person, but the person had made him angry and he had done something wrong. Now he was sorry about it but he had got to face reality.

[What had he done?]

Killed someone, of course.

[Woman looking in through half-open door]

Jane had lived in this dark, quiet house 20 miles from the nearest civilization for more than 10 years. She had been haunted by the fact that she hadn't treated her husband very well before his death. That is why she has formed ideas about the house and about reasons why vases fall over—the bulb goes out and books fall down. There were really quite logical explanations for these things. There has been a storm in the night. But Jane thinks of these happenings and connects them with the way she had treated her husband. She created problems for herself by doing this and makes her life a misery. She is scared to go out of the house. She doesn't like staying in the house. When she goes to sleep she is afraid of what will happen while she is asleep and what she will find when she wakes up. She is always ready to quickly turn round, but she finds nothing unusual. She just connects them and thinks about and worries about them as if they were connected with the way she had treated her husband.

CASE 2   Amy was referred to us because of her hand-washing compulsion and an intense preoccupation with dirt. She was a pale, thin, unhappy, anxious girl who, at 19, looked more like a 14-year-old. Her average intelligence as well as her clumsy unsteady gait may well have been due to brain damage at birth. She was grossly dependent on her mother, far in excess of anything warranted by either her physical or mental handicap. Indeed, the paucity of progressive forces was one of the most striking features in her whole development. We gained the impression that Amy hardly ever felt good about herself in any respect, and she seemed to share her parents' view—that she was far more mentally and physically defective than was actually the case. Such a view made it well-nigh impossible for these rather obsessional, intellectual, middle-class parents, in their concern, anxiety, shame, and guilt, to help Amy toward greater independence. Thus, her relationship to her mother remained extremely infantile. There were indications of some phallic-oedipal strivings, but it seemed unlikely that Amy ever reached oedipal phase dominance.

However, Amy had a sense of humor and could even laugh at herself. She could make friendly contacts—and did so in treatment. Although she occasionally showed some awareness of the feelings of others, her own wishes and needs had to come first. Her concerns and fears were for herself, not for her objects. Nevertheless, away from home, for instance, at day school, Amy was sometimes able to function better and her school attainments matched the level of her ability.

Amy's hand-washing compulsion began when she was sent to boarding school at the age of 16 upon the recommendation of the school authorities who thought that this might help her achieve greater independence. Until then the care of Amy's body had been entirely under her mother's control. When Amy, at the age of 16, was suddenly thrown on her own resources for the control of her impulses, especially her strong anal drives, she was unable to cope without symptom formation. Left to her own devices, she washed her hands until they were raw and bleeding.

When she returned home, after six months, the family was heavily involved in her toilet habits. She occupied the bathroom endlessly—wiping, washing, afraid of touching, wondering whether or not she was really clean or whether or not she had "done something." She persuaded her mother to keep wiping her bottom. She always expressed the great fear, first touched off by the Matron at boarding school, that she might smell. She kept an eagle eye on whether other people washed and when she was out in the street had eyes for nothing but dogs' dirt, horses' dirt, or birdlime, afraid she would get dirty and yet, perhaps, getting some gratification from the sight of it. Her endless performances in the bathroom and her constant preoccupation with doubts and conversations about these matters drove those around her to distraction and led to bitter disputes within the family. However, we do not think that her compulsions were based mainly on object-directed aggression. She seemed to defend mainly against forbidden, pleasurable aspects of her anal drives. It may be that the presence of her objects is needed to protect her against the temptation of anal masturbation.

Comparison of the Two Cases

Although these two cases show certain similarities, some of the differences are very striking. We have already pointed to the considerable disparity in intellectual endowment. When we turn to the acute onset of symptoms, we note definite precipitating factors. In each case a distinct step toward independence was demanded by the environment, but the character and quality of those steps were in other respects quite different. In Ron's case, a step toward token manhood was undertaken; and the reemergence of oedipal conflicts in puberty was brought into focus. Ron's being forced by his mother to banish his father from the Bar Mitzvah was a dramatic enactment of oedipal death wishes which may have been instrumental in precipitating the illness. In Amy's case, the onset of the washing compulsion was equally dramatic, and occurred on separation from the mother. Until this separation, the care of the child's body had been entirely the mother's responsibility and was under her firm control. For Amy, she had come to represent a major external agent in the fight against dirt. The fight against impulse had thus been contained in the context of the mother-child relationship; when that relationship was interrupted, the child was required to take over control without having the resources to do so. The level of object relationships in each case was therefore entirely different.

While Ron's obsessional symptoms disappeared within the first weeks of analytic treatment, this was not the case with Amy. But it should be remembered that Amy did not start treatment until 2½ years after the onset of her hand-washing compulsion.

Each child fought against dirt. Ron feared that dirt might damage and be dangerous to his objects, a preoccupation that therefore reflected important derivatives of his death wishes. His mother experienced the symptom as aggressively torturing. Amy also fought against dirt, but in her case there was no such murderous component. She was afraid only for herself. Although her objects experienced her repetitive washing and interminable questioning as an attack, this appeared to play no part in her motivation. The use of the object as an external defense against dirt and anal masturbation has already been indicated. Ron, on the other hand, made no such defensive use of his mother.

While the conversion hysteric makes the move from mind to body in the somatic dramatization of his conflicts, the obsessional neurotic mentally removes himself from the bodily sources of his conflicts, so that the disturbance appears predominantly in the intellectual sphere. This is seen at its most structured and at its clearest in the adult obsessional-ruminative disorders. It is true that in the initial phase of his disturbance, Ron showed a step toward such mentalization a particularly clear example of which was given by Ron in one of his interviews. Asked for three wishes, he stated two as follows: (1) He would like to know the commandment of the Creator. (2) He would like the Messiah all the Jews are waiting for to arrive soon, because if the Messiah arrives there will be *no* wars and the people will have only their *thoughts—no bodies anymore.*

It is also true that Ron's initial preoccupation with Talmudic law resembles the ruminations of the obsessional neurotic, but in his case this was conspicuously transient and did not endure much beyond the time taken for the assessment of his case. When he was taken into analysis these early intense preoccupations with Jewish law took on a *cultural* quality and lost their pathological character. The brief excursion of Ron's symptomatology into the mental sphere, with its concomitant attempt to hold in check the upsurge of pubertal forces, soon gave way to the intensive preoccupation with dirt and the fantasied danger to which his objects were exposed by his various bodily contents. It is noteworthy that he saw the danger stemming not from their supposedly contaminative character, but from indirect effects—that his mother would slip on his saliva or the dirt from his fingernails. We have also noted an attempt at displacement from the dangerous contents of his own body to the dangerous contents of animals such as birds or dogs. Amy's similar and unsuccessful attempt at displacement from her own body has been described. The closeness of the symptoms to the body underlines one further difference between the picture Amy presented and the compulsive hand-washing of the more classical cases: Amy tried, literally, to wash the *dirt* away; while the obsessional neurotic tries to wash away the *thought* of dirt.

While Amy had a superego, it had a primitive quality. She was unable to trust it and needed the reinforcement which her mother provided as an external ally in the fight against dirt. Ron's invocation of Talmudic law could be regarded as a step from the external source of authority and control toward an impersonal one, but his superego still lacked the fully internalized authority which makes the obsessional neurotic more independent of his objects as far as symptom formation is concerned. We also wondered whether the battle against dirt may precede the battle against aggression in symptoms of obsessional type.

When we look at the developmental aspects of Amy's disturbance and the way in which the influences of the mother-child relationship affected the development of her symptoms, we cannot fail to be struck by the impact of Amy's defectiveness on an ambitious and omnipotently controlling mother. The sense of bitter failure engendered in the mother was, in turn, reflected in her handling of the child and her attitude towards Amy—factors which served only to aggravate the disturbance and not to mitigate it. Ron's mother also had strong feelings of failure and guilt in relation to her handling of the boy, but, in contrast to Amy, Ron had no mental or physical handicaps.

The Other Cases

Of the five recent referrals we have mentioned, the remaining three, while otherwise differing in the details of their symptoms, all had compulsive hand-washing as a presenting clinical feature. We shall not attempt to describe these cases in detail, but all three showed a feature not present in the cases already discussed. They all appeared to take their mother's illness upon themselves—a tendency which lent the clinical picture the coloring of hypochondriasis.

In one of them, Len's compulsive washing rituals developed at 12½, also in the year of his Bar Mitzvah. The onset again was acute. There was a deterioration in his schoolwork and he started to wet the bed. Although there was no previous history of obsessional symptoms, he had been phobic at 4½. When the parents referred him, they could no longer stand the regime he imposed on them with his incessant washing. As in the other cases, this related directly to his need to avoid contamination with bodily products, and he spent hours washing himself after defecation or urination. He would wipe his bottom until it bled. In one respect, however, his concern showed some further displacement from the body and some degree of symbolization. This was reflected in his attitude to his camera which had to be wrapped in a plastic bag to protect it from contamination. This was thought to symbolize the skin and represent the fear of its penetration by dirt. He involved his mother in his symptoms and forced her to comply with his endless demands for washing his clothes.

Len's presenting picture included symptoms which had the misleading appearance of hypochondriasis. The boy complained of pain in the knees; although this had a mild physical basis, the intensity of his complaints were thought to be connected with the fact that somewhat earlier his mother had injured both knees in a car accident. He also complained of pain in the chest; again we thought it significant that the mother had had a breast biopsy for a suspected carcinoma. While at first sight this appeared to be an identification with the mother, in discussion a different explanation was suggested. It was as if the child offered his body to her illness in an attempt to protect the mother from it.

Our fourth case, Ned, also showed the coexistence of a seeming hypochondriasis and obsessional washing. His illness began dramatically after he had been hit in the chest by a football and he at once developed fears that his heart was damaged. We thought it significant that his mother had heart disease and that he knew that this had developed during her pregnancy with him. The wish to protect the mother by offering his own body to her illness appeared to be an important element in *his* symptom, as in the previous case; but his concern and overall anxiety about his body, and his rapidly developing fears of ravaging illness, were considerably greater.

His obsessional symptoms sprang from a fear that his mother had given him poisonous food or had contaminated the dishes on which it was served, by using soda. In this way the object was also involved in the cleansing process. Washing rituals occurred whenever he thought anyone might have touched him; this involved boys at school, and extended to doorknobs and cutlery which he thought either his mother or his sister might have touched. While we make only passing reference to him, we wish to emphasize one common feature in the onset of his illness and that of our first case, Ron. *His* obsessional symptoms, too, cleared up within the period of the diagnostic assessment; and when he came into analysis, the remaining symptomatic picture was that of fears, phobias, and the persisting somatic symptoms.

In our fifth case, Colin, compulsive washing began at the age of 10, and was accompanied by contamination fears. But, as in the previous case, some of the obsessional elements quickly diminished while the phobic ones increased.

Some aspects of *his* symptoms might also be related to his mother's illness, namely, her "secret" alcoholism. This may be an explanation of his unusual fear of contamination, namely, the fear of taking in drugs. He avoided long-haired people and junkies who he thought might possibly contaminate him with them. His constant fear of being unwittingly injected by drugs, or of breathing them in, bordered on the bizarre. His symptoms began suddenly when a girl at his school was thought to be taking drugs.

There were several features which *all* our patients had in common. We have already mentioned that none of our children was outstandingly bright and that they did not show the precocious ego development commonly seen in obsessional neurotics. On the contrary, some gave the impression of rather impoverished development. None of them seemed to have good feelings about themselves. They showed little by way of achievements and we were struck by the dearth of sublimation. Their social relationships were disturbed and they had few friends. At the time when their world ought to have been expanding, it was in fact contracting and they were becoming increasingly isolated. While they should have been 'gaining greater distance from their parents, they and their parents actually became even more closely enmeshed via the children's symptomatology. At least some of our children came from obviously obsessional households, but all the parents were equally trapped. Except in those conflicts with their parents which derived from their symptomatology, overt expressions of aggression tended to be inhibited in these children.

Discussion

Among the points which seemed relevant in these cases are: the sudden onset and, in some cases, the quick disappearance of symptoms; the pronounced and active involvement of the outside world which led to conflicts with their families; the defense against dirt itself; the lack of symbolization and intellectualization; and, in some cases, additional symptoms bearing a superficial resemblance to hypochondriasis.

Although we are aware that sudden or rapid changes in the disturbances of adolescents are not unusual, we have wondered whether the sudden onset of obsessional symptoms at an earlier age might be a characteristic feature of the type of disturbances with which we are concerned. The ages of our children ranged from 9 to 13, that is, late latency and prepuberty. This is somewhat later than the age Freud (1913) first described as typical for the onset of obsessional neurosis; namely, between 6 to 8 years.

In "A Study of the Mechanism of Obsessive-Compulsive Conditions" (1923), Greenacre described 86 adult patients and stated that they came for treatment between the ages of 16 and 40. Acute symptoms began most frequently between 21 and 25, but most of the patients gave a retrospective account of obsessions and compulsions beginning before puberty. As regards the onset of illness in children, Lewin (1948) states that while compulsive phenomena may occur in the third year, the neurosis usually begins in the latency period, between the fourth and twelfth years. Several of the cases referred to the Hampstead Clinic, which Nagera (1965) described, showed a "completely developed obsessional neurosis sometime between the ages of 9-12 years." In other words, the group of children recently referred to us does not differ from Nagera's with regard to age. What Nagera did *not* describe was the sudden onset of symptoms.

While in all our cases the sudden onset appeared to be related to a definite precipitating factor, the somewhat unexpectedly quick disappearance of these symptoms in some of the children also attracted our attention. We began to speculate on a possible link between a rapid onset of illness and an equally rapid amelioration of the obsessional features, even though such symptoms then gave way to others. We wondered whether this changeability of symptoms might give a further hint of the relative instability of the underlying psychic structure of these children, a point we have already made in the comparison between Amy and Ron.

The great dependency of our children on the object world, while characteristic of many childhood disturbances, is in sharp contrast to the true obsessional neurotic about whom Freud (1907) wrote:

> It is remarkable that both compulsions and prohibitions (having to do something and having *not* to do something) apply in the first instance only to the subject's solitary activities and for a long time leave his social behaviour unaffected. Sufferers from the illness are consequently able to treat their affliction as a private matter and keep it concealed for many years [p. 119].

We realize that such a fully developed obsessional neurosis is rare in childhood. In our cases the urge to fulfill the compulsive demands showed greater intrusion into the common social milieu and included the demand for participation by the objects. The obsessional symptoms could not be contained as "a private matter" but took the form of disturbing behavior which increasingly afflicted family life to the very borders of tolerance. A large measure of urgency in the referrals stemmed from the sudden eruption of the child's imposing and controlling behavior. While this was generally experienced by the family as an aggressive attack, it does not, of course, follow that the symptoms necessarily included aggressive motivation or intent.

We asked ourselves how these children related to their parents before the onset of symptoms. One of Amy's TAT stories suggested a great lack of communication and exchange in the relationship:

> Once upon a time there was a mother with a daughter and they lived alone in this house. While the mother was reading, the lovely girl was looking the other way. She was holding her doll and she was thinking about how it would be in fifteen years' time—whether she would still have as much pleasure as she had at first and she was thinking about that and her mother wasn't interested in her, she was reading the book. While she was thinking she wasn't doing anything; she was just thinking and her mother continued reading because she had to do that for school. She had to do the reading for teaching, so she read it.

The question arises whether, with the aid of the symptom, the children try to maintain an active relationship at a time when they feel a threat to it. Would such a use be a secondary one, an epinosic gain; or would it play a more primary part in symptom formation?

In diagnostic discussions the opinion was expressed that the child's dependence on the parents increased so much because the parents were exploited for defensive purposes. While we were often struck by the apparent collusion of the parents with the children's demands, Anna Freud suggested that such a collusion sprang from the parents' anxiety and fear of temper tantrums and sometimes even of the children's sadism. Certainly, noncompliance by the parents resulted in aggressive outbursts by the children. To some extent these were certainly due to the children's anxiety; yet, in some of the cases we may also have witnessed, in the child's control of the parents, a return of sadistic pleasure and anal aggression originally checked by defense.

This brings us to the theme of the defense against dirt itself. In all our cases dirt was avoided in a concrete way. Obsessional actions such as hand washing exceeded obsessional thinking. There was a notable lack of symbolization and intellectualization. When thinking *was* involved, it had a concrete quality and was largely about dirt itself. We also asked ourselves about the relation between the fight against dirt and the conflict about aggression. We noted that those children who feared they might be harmed by dirt did not fear that the same dirt might harm their objects. It is this which made us wonder whether, developmentally, defense against dirt may antedate defense against aggression and whether, in a girl like Amy, it was dirt, rather than aggression, which was originally defended against in her symptoms.

To what extent, in some of the children, is a preoccupation with dirt in this concrete sense related to a libidinal fixation, to distortion in ego development, perhaps attended with a particular immaturity in the object relationship? And how far, in certain cases, has aggression within this relationship been *reduced* to conflict about anality, rather than *preceded* by it, so that the objectionable feeling is replaced by an objectionable thing, namely, dirt, which is visible and can be avoided? However this may be, the link between the fight against dirt and the fight against aggression is exemplified by Ron's fear of harming his mother through causing her to slip on his saliva and excreta. However, in Ron's case, entry into the oedipal phase and the emergence of death wishes toward the father, led to regressive reactivation of conflict over the aggressive aspects of the anal phase, with consequent sympton formation on that level.

If, in some of our cases, the obsessional symptoms involve the mother in a sadistic and aggressively controlling way, then the reverse side of the coin may be seen, at least descriptively, in those of our cases which showed a pseudohypochondriasis in the child's unconscious offer of his own body to the mother's illness in order to protect her. If this interpretation is correct, it raises the fascinating question as to the extent to which, in one and the same child, one set of symptoms can show rather clearly the return of the repressed drive derivative, while a

coexistent symptom can reveal a more predominantly successful defensive aspect of the illness.

Further reflection led us to ask ourselves why the children
had such a great need to protect the mother. We conjectured
that a real danger to the mother's life, through accident or
illness, had so increased the threat of the children's death
wishes that the only way to protect her from these wishes was to
become ill in her place. We also considered a further view.
Becoming aware that a conflictual object has been damaged,
the child might believe that he had brought about this damage
by his secret omnipotent aggression. He then takes it over, so
that a fantasied crime is transformed into self-punishment.

So far we have tried to differentiate between children presenting with obsessional symptoms and those suffering from a
true obsessional neurosis. However, in all the present cases the
severity of the condition was such that the question of the
existence of an underlying psychosis could not be overlooked.
These doubts arose from a certain bizarre quality of the symptoms and from the fact that the child's fear of contamination
on delusional conviction, without, however, the total suspen-
sion of reality testing. These doubts persisted, even though
nearly all the children made quite a warm affective contact
during their interview, as Greenson pointed out in discussion.
Ned was an exception: he was far too anxious and inhibited to
display such warmth. We were not even certain what the
children were defending against: were the obsessional defenses
directed against increasing pubertal strivings or were they
keeping regression in check? We even had difficulty in knowing whether we were witnessing a breakdown of defenses or an
increase of defenses which would remain part of a permanent
structure. Thus, it is abundantly clear that, in spite of the use
of the Profile, we were left in many instances with numerous
unresolved questions about these children's psychopathology
and, particularly, about their prognosis. Ron, perhaps, is an
exception.

Such questions of pathology and prognosis are far from
academic, since they lead to the most important question of all:
what treatment is likely to benefit these children most? And if

they are taken into psychoanalytic treatment, what modifications of technique might one need to consider from the very beginning? Clearly, defense analysis has its dangers. Further, as we have emphasized, these children often use their objects for defensive purposes—a fact which led Anna Freud to suggest that this in itself presents "a grave danger to treatment, transference, and treatment alliance: when the adults around him cease to serve his defenses, the child may become very phobic of treatment."

When we came to write this paper, Anna Freud suggested that a more appropriate title than the one we had chosen might well be: "We thought we understood obsessional neurosis, but after studying five patients with obsessional symptoms we realize that we don't." We thus remain in the same position as Sigmund Freud when he said, in 1926: "Obsessional neurosis is unquestionably the most interesting and repaying subject of analytic research. But as a problem it has not yet been mastered" (p. 113).

7

STANLEY WISEBERG, CLIFFORD YORKE, and PATRICIA RADFORD

Aspects of Self Cathexis in "Mainline" Heroin Addiction: A Preliminary Report

A critical review of the psychoanalytic literature on drug addiction by one of us (Yorke, 1970) firmly established that psychoanalytic contributions to our understanding of the diagnostic status of serious addiction was marred by confusion, ambiguity, and contradiction.[1] Obvious problems included matters of definition, but the anomalies encountered went far beyond such questions. Yorke, therefore, concluded his review as follows:

> A glance at the headings of Anna Freud's Adult Diagnostic Profile highlights better than anything else the existing gaps in our knowledge. How would the sections on self-cathexis, on . . . narcissism, look in a diagnostic profile of these cases? There is no way round the fact that a psychoanalytic diagnosis is a metapsychological diagnosis. It seems, therefore, logical to apply the diagnostic profile to cases of addiction at the stage of initial investigation, although one must be prepared to find that this procedure poses further questions which can perhaps only be answered in analysis [p. 156f.].

In the light of this conclusion, we embarked on a series of Profile studies of "mainline" heroin addicts (Radford,

From the Group for the Study of "Mainline" Heroin Addiction.

[1] The relevant bibliography reported in that paper is not repeated here, and subsequent additions to the literature have not called for modifications in the conclusions.

99

Wiseberg, and Yorke, 1972). In this preliminary report we gave a fairly full account of the investigative method we had adopted. We stated:

> It became evident that the [Diagnostic] Profile provided a standardized structure for the fullest possible assessment of the patient within the limits of the available data. Since this structure is known and reproducible by psychoanalytically trained clinical research workers anywhere, the Profile can be checked and rechecked wherever the original data are available. Furthermore, practiced users of the Profile should have a high standard of consistency from case to case; and there should, in addition, be reliable comparisons between the work of one group of investigators and another. . . .
>
> It seems to us that it is precisely these considerations which make the Profile especially suited to the evaluation of groups of patients who, from a descriptive point of view, are commonly classified together but whose nosological status otherwise remains uncertain [p. 158f.].

Our current Profile studies were based on detailed social histories and psychiatric reports derived from extended interviews carried out by ourselves. To minimize the number of variables we confined our pilot investigation to 10 subjects who were regularly "mainlining" with heroin, whether or not they used additional drugs. All were seriously addicted to their drug to a point at which their craving for it and their need to procure it were for each the major priority; and all were physiologically as well as psychologically dependent on it. All were members of an inpatient unit for the treatment of addiction on therapeutic community lines. All had been withdrawn from drugs for some weeks before they were seen, though one or two had occasional "slips." We confined ourselves to those cases in which an independent early history was available—a measure which further restricted the range of patients assessed. We realize that, had we restricted our studies to addicts serving prison sentences, for example, our findings might well have been different; but in our earlier report we have stated the reasons why the limitations of our selection criteria may not be too serious as long as they are stated and kept in mind.

In this paper we have confined ourselves to certain aspects of self cathexis and have chosen to illustrate these with three vignettes from the 10 cases of our pilot study.

Case 1

Gianetta was 23 years old at the time of her assessment. Rescued by her mother, a few weeks before our contact with her, from conditions of squalor and dereliction, she was so horrified by her own deterioration that she underwent a voluntary withdrawal without any supervision before deciding to seek medical help.

Gianetta was a dramatically elegant and strikingly good-looking red-head. Her well-groomed appearance was only slightly marred by a degree of jaundice occasioned by syringe hepatitis. She was lively and articulate, and of superior intelligence. She was pleasantly relaxed and enjoyed the interviews.

Gianetta was a highly skilled call girl, chess player, and dancer. She had sophisticated tastes and liked good living; and in spite of a working-class background, she was at home in all kinds of circles. She mixed with highly educated, successful, and eminent people, earning their admiration and deference.

Gianetta was the child of a handsome, well-dressed Irish mother and an alcoholic Italian father. She, the first, only, and unplanned child of the marriage, was a robust and lusty infant who quickly thrived. She walked and talked early in her second year. Toilet training was achieved abnormally quickly; she never regressed; and both mother and child took pride in her cleanliness.

Gianetta's early development took place against a background of violent scenes and sustained drunkenness, but when she was 18 months old, there was a temporary reduction in the father's drinking and he began to enjoy the child. When the pubs closed he would bring his friends to the house, fetch his daughter from her bed, and show her off to them. She would be the center of admiration—an event that may have been important for her subsequent narcissistic organization.

However, the drinking and family strife soon reached unbearable proportions. Gianetta developed temper tantrums, nightmares, and sleeping difficulties. The mother slept with the

child, ostensibly to protect her from her father; but this was
continued after the marriage broke up when the child was 4.
Gianetta then missed her father intensely.

The mother now had to work and left the child in the care of
relatives. When Gianetta was 7 her mother moved into a flat of
her own, and the little girl became a "latchkey" child. She
would return from school at 3:30 and make herself and her
mother a cup of tea; the mother's cup awaited her return two
hours later.

After a year, the mother remarried. The stepfather displaced
Gianetta from her mother's bed. His two children deprived her
of her mother's attention. Furthermore, the stepfather was
tyrannical and physically cruel. When Gianetta was 13, her
mother discovered that, in spite of academic success, Gianetta
had truanted and had repeatedly forged notes and imperson-
ated her mother on the telephone to explain her absence.
Actually, she was working as a paid hostess at a gambling club.

In this way Gianetta's aberrant sexual development, which
had begun with seduction by an uncle at the age of 3 and
continued throughout childhood, took a further step with her
physical maturation. She left school at the earliest opportunity.
She became pregnant, married, and abandoned the baby to its
father who left her. Soon she became a wealthy call girl with
handsome apartments in London and Rome, where she in-
dulged the varied and perverse tastes of her clients. She had a
number of sexual friendships with both men and women, in
which she showed her predilection for humiliating and punish-
ing her objects. For example, she said: "I felt very sexy. I
bought a couple of penny canes. I tied Sam up and tied his
penis in a little bag and beat him. This was very exciting for
both of us. It gave me a feeling of power."

Gianetta started on cannabis in her early teens, soon trans-
ferring to LSD. She began to lose some of her drive and was
increasingly unable to follow her career as a call girl. Her
personal and sexual relationships deteriorated. After she
moved on to heroin, via barbiturates and amphetamines, she
abandoned sexual activity altogether. Once she began "main-
lining" she was quickly "hooked" and her only surviving interest was in getting and maintaining drug supplies. She lost

her money and was soon living "rough" with the "junkies" she despised.

It cannot be doubted that Gianetta's narcissistic organization was highly pathological, but she has real pride in her appearance and her dress, though this betrayed a compensatory and phallic quality. The sources of this pride included an identification with a handsome and well-groomed mother, and the admiration of her father and his friends which must have contributed to her self-esteem and self-regard and to her pleasurable expectations of shining in society. The cathexis of her mental self and her ego skills was high, but this too had a compensatory quality. Gianetta basically had a deficient libidinal cathexis of herself, so that she was unhappy and self-contemptuous. Her continuing need for external narcissistic supplies could be seen in the fact that she was at her best only when she felt herself cared for or approved of by a maternal figure. She could not be alone and had not slept by herself for 10 years. Even at the age of 3 she took money from her father's till to pay her friends to stay with her.

Her attitude to her body was fundamentally ambivalent and she showed strong penis envy. Her degradation of herself in her profession as a call girl was significant. This seemed to us to indicate an aggressive cathexis of the self as well as a diminished libidinal endowment. But she could also use her aggression in the service of her personality.

With regard to the relative distribution of libido between self and objects, we can say that objects were not important to Gianetta except as the means to an end. Among these ends were: being provided and cared for; furthering social climbing; obtaining admiration and attention; controlling, debasing, and torturing; and obtaining masturbatory experiences. She exploited her partners' sexual needs and did not grant them importance in their own right. Since her object relationships gave a strong indication of her dependency needs and existed largely to be made use of, they may in this respect have had the status of *transitional objects*.

Drugs, at first sight, may have had a *similar* status, but they did not increase her self-esteem. They were used for sexual gratification but she could not take them when she was alone.

Equally she could masturbate only in the presence of a partner who was required to masturbate simultaneously. Her relations to drugs and the syringe progressively replaced object relations until they had virtually taken over. Masturbation was displaced to fixing. "I think the needle and syringe are as important as the drug. I like to flush a great deal and I do it over and over again. I am sure this is sexual. It's like masturbation. I always tried to put off the orgasm as long as possible. If I felt one coming on, I would stop and then start again and swear by something holy." With the patient as both subject and object, a narcissistic system was established which was never quite complete since she still needed the company of a partner.

The sexual gratification was accompanied by an aggressive attack on both the bodily and mental self and was partly mediated via the superego. It was in the drug-taking phase that the aggressive cathexis of the self took the upper hand. Later she recalled with horror her filth and deterioration; and she cried with shame when she told the psychiatrist how she found a flea in her hair when she was sharing a room with "junkies."

Problems of Self-Esteem

At this stage it seems appropriate to comment briefly on these patients' self-esteem; the early cathexis which they received from their families; and certain contributions which aggression makes to the level of self-esteem. Our report is, therefore, restricted and tentative, but does, we think, highlight certain similarities and differences to be found among this small number of addicts.

In assessing self-esteem we were able to draw on a wide range of reasonably consistent information, from both patients and their relatives, covering much of the addicts' history, so that it was possible to make an assessment of the level of self-esteem before, during, and after the drug-taking phase. Where anomalies existed, the genetic origins of these could often be detected. In general, the patients' habitual level of self-esteem appeared constant over many years, if not from childhood, leaving aside any changes which had taken place during severe drug-taking phases. These general characteristics apart, it was the great variability in degree and quality of esteem between the different subjects that was most striking.

With one possible exception all our patients had experienced, either from early childhood or from puberty, a deficiency of self-esteem which included, in some degree, one or more of the following features: an impaired sense of well-being, a lack of confidence, prevailing feelings of inferiority, and an inability to make reasonable use of their various skills and personality attributes. However, some patients (for example, Paul, who is discussed below) were not particularly incapacitated by their views of themselves, at least not until advanced stages of addiction supervened; and after withdrawal of drugs, they could, at least for a period, regain this level. In others, self-esteem was so seriously impoverished that they felt unequipped for life at almost any level (for example, see Ronald). While we claim no statistical provenance for the observation, it is worth commenting that our cases fall into two roughly equal groups: one in which self-esteem is severely impaired, and the other in which it is only mildly or moderately impaired. We do not wish to imply that any such impairment is the prerogative of addicts.

Looking at the cathexis which the patients have received in early life from their parents and other members of their families, we find that, in general, members of the group with very low self-esteem were poorly or ambivalently cathected by their families; while those who fell into the group whose self-esteem was not so impaired had received more constant and sustained love and appreciation from at least one parent and sometimes from both. We are aware that early parental cathexis, however important, is not specific for any particular outcome in personality development.

There were a few seeming anomalies. In one of our cases, the child had been intensely cathected by his parents, though perhaps narcissistically, but throughout his life his self-esteem was unusually low. This is one of the reasons why we have chosen him for more detailed illustration. In another case, the child had been clearly unwanted by the mother, but he was nevertheless able to take a good view of himself and showed considerable interest in appearance and achievement. It is true, however, that he was much wanted by his father, though the history did not indicate that the closeness of the paternal relationship was sufficient to counteract adverse maternal influence. Perhaps this serves to remind us that there are, in all such cases, imponderables at the diagnostic stage which subsequent analysis might help us understand better, a privilege denied us in all but one of our cases. (Not that we suggest that many of these cases are analyzable.)

The drugs our patients used are undeniably dangerous. This brings us to a question asked by many: "To what extent is the use of the drug a motivated attack on the self?" After all, the possibility remains that, in some instances, the apparent attack on the self may be coincidental rather than sought.

The concept of basic aggressive cathexis of the self is problematical and our views on it have yet to be clarified. However this may be, it is well known that self-attack may come about in a number of different ways. In some, it appears to have a defensive function and has served to protect the object from aggression. In other cases, guilt and the need for punishment are powerful factors; and moral masochism may also play an important role. We also have in mind cases in which there may be attacks on parental identifications. Yet again, attacks on the body as a source of unwanted instinctual urges may also be a feature in certain addictive cases. Lastly, we must consider the possibility that the use of drugs may be resorted to in order to punish the object. When one of our patients started using Chinese heroin—after a row with his mother—he did so with the thought: "I hate you, I know best:" He added: "If I destroy myself, I knew it would upset my parents." The fact that self-attack may have multiple meanings in the same patient is shown by his remark: "When I was on drugs and when I was furious with my parents, I left the house in a temper, took my father's car, and although I was not insured, I drove violently for 100 miles up the motorway." He added that when he returned, he drove very slowly and carefully, but was compelled to report himself to the police.

It is often difficult to discern, at the stage of diagnostic assessment, which of these forms of aggressive self-attack may have been operative. We have, however, enough evidence to show that there is a wide variety in the meaning and use of aggressive attacks on the self in these patients. As in so many other matters, there seems to be a wide scatter and little uniformity.

In concluding this section we pose the question: "Why do people *use dangerous* drugs?" While the answer can only be found, if at all, by full metapsychological assessment, we would emphasize the possible relevance to the addict of any changes in self cathexis in self perception under the drug. What changes may the addict try to effect?

The drugs seem to have no consistent pharmacological effect on self-esteem, and it is in any event difficult to distinguish between psychological and pharmacological effects.

It seems to us that if the use of these drugs boosted self-esteem, this might well be felt by some to outweigh the dangers, especially so by those who have a defect in reality testing, however circumscribed, or whose egos are weak in other respects. However, in some of our cases there were no indications that the use of heroin had any such effect. In others, an apparent gain in self-esteem did not necessarily come about through the experience of the drug as an external source of narcissistic supply. There are other ways in which its use can raise self-esteem. Such a gain could arise through the modification of certain aspects of superego functioning. Some patients attempt to win the esteem of peer groups who use drugs by following their example. In yet other cases, self-esteem can be increased through changes in the defensive organization or by a redistribution of drive energy. One of our patients who disliked his aggressive self image said: "Until I took up drugs I had very poor control of my violent feelings. They would burst out all over the place. Since I have been taking drugs, I have felt much more at ease—I just don't get so aggressive." Yet another patient who, before taking drugs, showed such a severe timidity and inhibition of aggression that he was unable to use any adequate degree of aggressive energy to further normal adaptation, found that when he was under the influence of heroin without being completely "stoned," he could be constructively forceful. Other patients whose anxieties had been aroused by their libidinal urges found their libido

sufficiently damped down by drug taking to obviate these anxieties; and when their sexuality was a source of shame, the
taking of drugs heightened their self-esteem and feeling of
well-being.

It is also clear that many addicts take drugs for reasons other
than an attempted boost of self-esteem. Many take drugs for
kicks, for sexual gratification, and for these persons the "buzz"
is what really matters. Others who feel particularly miserable or
wretched and who are in some respects close to despair take
drugs for the feeling of Nirvana that they provide; under the
influence of heroin they no longer care. This was the case in
one of our woman patients about whose future we feel especially pessimistic; we fear that she will commit suicide, either
directly or indirectly, through her drug taking.

Other possible reasons for drug taking include the furthering of changes in the perception of the self and its relation to
the outer world so that the ego is presented with a more
acceptable self-image. Other writers have discussed this point.
There are also patients whose increased well-being appears to
be achieved via a drug-assisted withdrawal into an acceptable
fantasy world.

We shall illustrate these points with additional clinical examples.

Case 2

We begin with a boy whose self-esteem was severely impoverished. Ronald, 19 years old, was a dark, slightly built boy
with a long acne-scarred face, whose manner was shy and
diffident, though he had a good deal of childish appeal. Most
people felt protective toward him. He was noticeably careful
not to appear to be making any demands, and this seemed to
disguise a great wish for dependence. His range of affect was
limited; in particular, there seemed little conviction in his
condemnation of his addiction and misdemeanors. His appearance and manner were not in keeping with his fairly privileged
middle-class background. There was a predominant and fairly
constant mood of mild depression, with occasional flashes of
humor which only increased the effect of pathos.

Ronald was the first child and only son of orthodox Jewish parents, who said that he was a much wanted, though unplanned child. In spite of this, we had the impression that the parents' professed love for their child was mainly narcissistic, and apparently was not expressed in their actual behavior to the child. Both parents were highly successful business people who were ambitious both for themselves and their children. They expected Ronald to continue their progress in climbing the social ladder. From the beginning, the mother imposed her own standards of behavior on the child; she demanded politeness, cleanliness, and conformity. Her attitude to his feeding typified her later handling of the child. She put him on solids at the age of 4 months and persisted in her efforts in spite of the child's adverse reaction; when he continued to protest, she took away the bottle. Feeding difficulties became firmly established, and by the age of 18 months, Ronald's health was in danger. Even then, the mother felt unable to make concessions. She still tried to enforce her own standards. The father said the slightest sign of messiness, e.g., the dropping of a pea, caused his wife to lose her temper with the violence of a hurricane.

Although the parents were aware of the child's total lack of satisfaction, they were unable to modify their attitude. They were constantly critical of the child; and increasingly, Ronald felt incapable of meeting their demands or coping with them from his own resources.

As his childhood progressed, Ronald approached all his endeavors with the expectation of failure, though he always hoped that some magical move on the mother's part would bring about some wished-for change. For example, although, from puberty onward, he was failing drastically at school and left without any academic credentials, he could still cling to the belief that because his mother had said that he would go to university, that was where he would ultimately find himself.

This belief in the mother's magic extended to the use of medicines. Ronald expected every ill to be cured by the medicaments he always demanded. When, at puberty, his feelings of inferiority in relation to his peers were increased by the physical disfigurement of severe acne, his doctor gave him phenobarbitone. Ronald then started taking hashish and amphetamines, and for the first time in his life experienced positive feelings of self-esteem. He said, "I had always regarded myself as relegated to a back seat. I admired my friends' power and activity. But drugs gave me a stronger personality." He said that now his friends admired his power and deferred to him.

Ronald started with hash at 13 years; he progressed through physeptone and methedrine; and by 16 he was "main-lining" heroin. During the course of this escalation, he had taken part in "breaking and entering" to gain acceptance in a group of delinquent addicts. Thus, despite the gain in his self-esteem induced by drugs, he still needed external approval. It was these activities which finally took him to court; and as a result of a probation order, he found himself a patient in the Drug Addiction Unit.

It will be clear that this brief history is selective, and that we have concentrated on those aspects which appear to have a bearing on Ronald's self-cathexis. He received little loving in childhood, and he failed to develop any adequate means whereby he could love or respect himself until he began to take drugs. He was therefore totally reliant on external sources of narcissistic supplies. Feeling so despicable and unlovable, he could not believe that anyone could really care for him. He felt he had fallen far below his parental ideals. In terms of both his bodily and his mental self he saw himself as an ugly, acne-ridden, useless failure. He had difficulties using his endowments—such as his intelligence—in the service of his personality and his relationships with others.

He tried to gain acceptance through compliance. With his parents he attempted to be the "good, conforming" boy; in the same way, with his peers, he was whatever they wanted him to be—even a delinquent lending them his mother's car for their robberies. This chameleonlike quality seemed to stem from his only self-ideal—to be the loved, wanted child, getting approval from anyone by any means. This basic need seems to have hindered any full internalization of other standards.

Ronald's aggression was not at the service of his personality. Indeed, from childhood onward, he had been terrified of any aggressive manifestation. He said, "If someone raised a voice, I thought there was going to be a fight, so I always agreed with everything. I thought anyway that they must be in the right." His aggression was equally inhibited in the service of his sexual drive. He said that no matter how much he loved someone, he could not get involved in any violent feelings; he would have to leave them. He described an occasion when he was talking to his girlfriend. A boy on a motorbike offered her a ride which she accepted. Ronald did nothing. He told the psychiatrist: "I would never fight for a girl." He was also physically impotent and later blamed this on his fixing; but he still preferred the use of his syringe to sexual activity.

Ronald was one of our patients for whom drugs undoubtedly boosted self-esteem. Under their influence, he was able to take a great interest in clothes and his capacity to dress well now afforded him much pride. "I became a leader of Carnaby Street fashion." Under the influence of drugs he felt at ease in the company of his peers. "The drugs made me feel ten feet tall."

His ways of coping with his aggression changed under drugs. Inhibitions were lessened. He became openly sadistic toward his parents, and for the first time in his life he began to make demands on them. The worry he caused them by his constant absences was deliberate. As for his peers, he increased his feeling of power and domination over the group by pushing drugs on them. There can be no doubt that, for Ronald, drugs were both magical and potent. Under their influence, he was able to use his intelligence much more effectively; but he did so mainly to find increasingly sophisticated ways of obtaining supplies and acquiring quite fantastically accurate knowledge of drugs and their various properties.

It is of some interest that Ronald's attitude to his syringe bordered on idolatry. In the course of one of his interviews, he said: "I think the syringe itself and the needle were a stronger factor than the drugs; and people joked about how I carried it around in a little glass case, as if it were something to be worshiped.

In spite of the improvement in his self-esteem, and in spite of the more uninhibited display of aggression, Ronald was not able to use the latter constructively and he was failing at his work. The drugs did not help him to find any real or stable relationship; nor did they help to reduce the severity of the critical aspects of his uneven superego. Even with drugs, he continued to feel extremely guilty. He reached the point where, in spite of his apparent success with his peers, he felt that his activities were wrong; and at moments of such critical realization, he would start to cry, feel badly about himself, but could not avoid the conviction that there was no alternative but to carry on along the pathway he had set himself.

Case 3

We now briefly describe the case of Paul, which from the standpoint of self-esteem and self-regard contrasts sharply with Ronald. Paul was a young man of 26, of average athletic build and with dark and rather lanky hair. Compared with his contemporaries, he was square in both dress and manner. In the interviews, he was easy, relaxed, and friendly, with something of a man-to-man quality. At times, his attitude was mildly histrionic. The charming talker, described in an interview by his mother, was easily recognizable.

Paul was the second son of middle-class parents. His father was an accountant who gave all his spare time to acting. His mother was a manageress at a delicatessen. The pregnancy was unwanted, but as soon as the baby was born, the mother's great pleasure in feeding rapidly led her to accept and love the baby. Feeding was a mutual gratification to the nursing couple. This shared satisfaction continued throughout his childhood and adult life, and he even enjoyed her food when he was on drugs.

Paul reached his childhood milestones early. By 18 months he was a fluent talker. One aspect of his personality, which his mother described as the con man, could be detected at an early age—"he could talk himself out of anything." In general, he made satisfactory progress in all areas, until he came into competition with his academically successful older brother. No one expected Paul to compete with his brother successfully, and although he obtained a place at his brother's grammar school, it seemed that his fear of competitive rivalry forced him to take up an attitude that was totally different from John's.

Unlike the latter's industrious application, Paul was rebellious and inattentive. He soon became a leading member of a somewhat delinquent group, and took pleasure in being different from his "goody-goody" brother. He became involved in a series of minor delinquencies which culminated, at 15, in an attack on a school prefect who was beaten up and had to be treated in a hospital. Paul showed no guilt about this incident.

The headmaster was not, it seems, displeased when Paul left school at the first opportunity. He took a job as a mechanical apprentice in which the work was somewhat tedious and repetitive. But he found his workmates pleasant and considered the work a bit of a giggle; in describing this period, he added that he could tolerate anything. It was about this time that he first became interested in pot. This was not, however, seen as a means of relieving tedium. Paul was not without interests; for example, he had a sophisticated understanding of jazz. Under the influence of pot he felt that every note sounded clearer, and said, "From the first, it felt as if waves of pleasure were floating through my body, and I could see no reason why I should not go on repeating the experience. I thought drug taking was rather glamorous and dangerous." This daredevil approach nevertheless concealed a sense of guilt. When he found himself a girlfriend who resembled his mother, he had to tell her about his drug taking, even though he knew she would rid herself of him. It is of interest that he was fond of this girl, respected her, and had no sexual relations with her; his sexual experiences were carried on at the same time with a denigrated female object, a 36-year-old woman.

He gave up his job and went to work with his brother in the theater, but finding himself once more in competition with his brother, he failed lamentably. He decided he would fulfill a lifelong ambition of traveling to the West Indies. He thoroughly relished all his experiences aboard and ashore during the trip, which he shared with a flamboyant male shipmate. At each meal they distended their stomachs with massive quantities of chianti and spaghetti. His exploits led him to demand money from the Consulate, which recouped from his parents.

On his return to England, he obtained a position in a travel agency. His travel experiences and his gift of the gab made him a great success. He worked well and with enjoyment and was soon on the promotion ladder. By this time, however, he was hooked on heroin and was also taking methedrine and cocaine. The consequent instability in mood and activity affected his work and led him to seek admission to an inpatient unit. He was proud that his job was kept open for him, but felt that his addiction was a blow to his self-esteem. "My self-respect is important to me," he said.

No one will be surprised from this brief account that we estimate Paul to have a high libidinal self cathexis in comparison with the rest of the group. Before drugs he had considerable self-esteem and self-regard, feeling pride in himself and his achievements. He expected to be liked and enjoyed fellowship. He had always had regard for his bodily self; his appearance had always been important to him and he was dressed in the square conservative manner in keeping with his picture of himself as a pleasant, hardworking chap.

His aggression was within the ego's control, was used in the service of sublimations, and in seeking gratification. It also served his limited sexual activity. At least before his addiction there was no evidence that aggression was turned against the self. He avoided overt aggression toward men by identification with them. His ego ideals were twofold, reflecting the two aspects of his father. He liked to see himself as the square, stable, hardworking husband supporting a stable home; and he got sufficiently close to this ideal in appearance, manner, and above all in his work record to afford himself some satisfaction. In his experiences as a traveler and his associated fantasies, he emulated a flamboyant aspect of his father, expressed in the latter's hobby of acting.

Paul's failure to compete with his brother reflected an area of lessened self-esteem. It was also apparent in his rivalry for his mother's love, which we believe still contributed to his continued dependence on both parents. Even at the age of 26, he said, "If either of my parents died, I would die; life without them would be impossible." This oedipal conflict was also illustrated by his comment about his admired girlfriend whom he forced to give him up: "I did not feel worthy of the love of a good woman." He did, however, feel worthy of the favors of a denigrated woman, 15 years older than he, of whom he said: "I just went to her for pills and sex."

His self-esteem was regulated by the love, caring, and feeding he received from his objects, by his satisfaction in his work achievements, and by his pleasure in his fantasy, much of which he could carry into activity. His oral character was apparent.

There was little change in self cathexis when Paul was on drugs. He said: "Drugs gave me more energy, helped me to concentrate better, to be patient and more tolerant with people and to enjoy my work even more." But, as he indicated, he had all these abilities to a considerable degree before his addiction. Even at the height of his addiction, he continued to care for his body. He never looked sloppy or neglected, and he protected himself as much as he could from the drugs' dangerous effects by the great care he took in administering them. When his addiction interfered grossly with his work, he sought medical aid. "I do not want to be a slave to drugs. I have already destroyed too much of the life I like."

Drugs did, however, provide him with additional sensual gratification and excitement. He participated with a drug-taking group in bizarre experiences in a room decorated with fake spiders and psychedelic prints, where the aberrant sensual pleasures were enhanced by the administration of electric shocks. Even here he withdrew when he felt he was harming himself.

Drugs might thus, in a limited way, have helped to increase his self-esteem in the area of competitiveness in which he was vulnerable by allowing him to vie with his father in flamboyance. And as he said, they played into his sensual needs.

Conclusions

The most striking feature in the comparison of our cases is the lack of uniformity in the area of self cathexis. While this does not preclude the possibility of common factors and characteristics in areas we have yet to examine in detail, our preliminary impression is that the range and variety of disturbance may prove equally striking.

It is of course possible, as our examination of self-esteem in these cases suggests, that certain loose groupings may emerge; for example in the degree to which patients make use of drugs as external sources of narcissistic supplies.

These considerations suggest the possibility that the variability *between* the cases may reflect the disparities of psychic structure and functioning *within* each individual case. Whether or not this reflects a failure of the synthetic function of the ego during adolescent development, with a consequent lack of integration between disparate parts of the personality, remains an open question.

In this connection we would emphasize that, in all our cases, drug taking began in adolescence; while this may apply only to our selected sample, we have the impression that although the onset of drug taking does occur in latency and prepuberty, onset at adolescence is most common. This raises the question whether the process of adolescence forces the ego to find a solution which is in some respects syntonic, yet at the same time also disintegrative. Our material does not permit us to answer this question. Similarly, we feel that we still have a great deal to learn about the possible relationship between self-esteem regulation on the one hand, and the constructive use of aggression on the other.

In this paper we have chosen to discuss a few selected questions from the multitude which arise in the study of these baffling cases.

8

THOMAS FREEMAN

The Use of the Profile Schema
for the Psychotic Patient

The purpose of this paper is to give an account of the ways in
which a Profile schema can be used to examine and evaluate
the clinical phenomena which appear at the onset and during
the course of the different kinds of psychotic illness.

The Profile Schema

In common with the Profile schemata for child and adult
patients suffering from neuroses and allied disorders the
schema for the psychotic patient has as its aim a metapsychological assessment of the clinical manifestations. The
schema is designed to provide the means for classifying and
evaluating the phenomena, to reveal the extent to which the
patient's personality has been subject to dissolution, and to
gauge the developmental maturity of that personality as it was
prior to the illness. Schemata may be completed at the onset of
an illness, when the illness is well established, in remission, at
relapse after remission, and in chronicity.

The first three sections of the schema comprise the reason
for referral, the description of the patient, family background,
and personal history. Section IV deals with "Possibly Significant
Environmental Circumstances" and therefore requires some
interpretation of the observable data.

Section V of the schema presents the drive situation obtaining during the psychosis. The libidinal drives are assessed first
with regard to their quality. A distinction is made between the

<hr>

From the Group for the Study of Adult Psychosis.

117

clinical phenomena which spring from libido which has re-
verted to its original instinctual state and those which arise
from libido which has retained its sublimated condition. The
way in which the patient relates to others—whether at the level
of need satisfaction or object constancy—will depend on the
predominance of one or other form of the libido and the
presence or absence of a defense organization.

The libido must also be assessed in terms of its distribution
between self, real objects, and delusional object representations. A wide range of phenomena extending from inaccessibil-
ity and disinterest to a preoccupation with a delusional reality
can be categorized within the concept of abnormalities of libido
distribution.

Aggression is also assessed according to its quality, objects,
and aims. Special attention is given to the nature of its relations
with the libido and to the degree to which it may manifest itself
autonomously.

In the sixth or ego section a description is given of the
symptoms and behavioral disorders which result from the
disorganization of speech, thinking, perception, memory, and
motility. Next, with the introduction of the status of the defense organization and the delineation of the danger situations
to which the ego reacted, both the dynamic and the economic
aspects of the clinical phenomena are brought to the fore. The
ego section concludes with a description of the predominant
affects and their relationship to drive activity and defense.

Disorders of the superego are placed within the ego section
of the schema. The superego may be inactive as occurs in
mania; it may be externalized as in paranoid states and in
severe depressions. The schema enables connections to be
established between superego function on the one hand and
the drive derivatives on the other hand. When the drives are
characterized by oral-sadistic tendencies, a similar orientation
will appear in the superego irrespective of whether it retains its
internalized status or has been externalized.

The next four sections of the schema (VII-X) present some
difficulty because in contrast to the earlier sections their completion is more dependent on inferences made from the observable phenomena and on reports obtained from nurses,

social workers, ancillary medical staff, and relatives. These sections have been drawn up first, to portray the kinds of regressions and forms of disorganization which have led to the clinical phenomena; second, to describe those acquired and constitutional influences, as reflected in the drives and the ego, which resulted in fixations during infancy and childhood; third, to present the kinds of conflicts operative in the psychosis—whether they are external, internalized, or internal. Consideration of conflicts leads to the tenth section which deals with the status of the patient's personality prior to the illness. Here information is sought concerning the extent to which the libido and the ego reached or approached their optimal development. Sections VII-X are entitled: "Assessment of Regressions and Possible Fixations;" "Results of Ego and Drive Disorganization;" "Assessment of Conflicts;" "Prepsychotic Personality."

It is essential to emphasize that when a Profile is completed on the basis of only a short acquaintance with the patient the material comprising the content of these last four sections must be regarded as provisional and in the nature of hypotheses. It is only later when further information is available from memories recalled by the patient or repeated by him with the analyst and with others with whom he is in immediate contact that a sound basis can be obtained for the metapsychological assessment of the psychotic attack.

The Use of the Schema

The schema, by virtue of its comprehensive format, is a suitable instrument with which to study some of the problems presented by the psychoses. In designating the schema an instrument, it must be remembered that Anna Freud et al. (1965) have pointed out that it "would be a grave misunderstanding . . . if the Profile were treated as a questionnaire, if it were allowed to dominate the interviewer's attitude during diagnostic examination . . . . What the Metapsychological Profile sets out to be is of a completely different order —namely, a framework for the analyst's thinking, and a method to organize findings after they have been elicited,

assimilated, and digested by him" (p. 10f.). With these considerations in mind, the schema has been used in studies of the
course and outcome of psychoses, of symptomatology and
classification, and in clinical research.

COURSE AND OUTCOME Psychoses which begin in late
adolescence or early in adult life and which are characterized
by paranoid syndromes do not ' necessarily follow the same
course or have the same outcome. In some, there is a continuing mental disintegration which leads either to a volitional and
affective defect or to a profound withdrawal, negativism, and
self-neglect. In others, there are remissions of varying degrees
of completeness. Only rarely do such cases end in states of
deterioration.

When paranoid syndromes appear between the ages of 25
and 50 years cases differ once again with regard to both course
and outcome. In patients who are married a complete remission of the illness frequently takes place, although there are
some where the paranoid complex becomes fixed, with the
illness passing into a state of chronicity. At the onset of all these
psychoses, whether it be in an adolescent or adult, in a single or
married person, the paranoid symptom complexes alone give
no indication as to the eventual course and outcome.

When we compare Profiles of such cases with one another,
we discern differences which can be related to the course of the
illness. The libidinal state differs from one case to the next not
only with respect to its quality and intensity but also with
regard to distribution. In cases where the psychosis has ended
in deterioration a severe permanent disorder of libido distribution may be inferred. The cathexis of real objects has been
almost entirely abandoned in favor of a cathexis of the self.
Sufficient cathexis of real objects remains in order to achieve
the fulfillment of needs. The outward manifestations of these
inner changes is a state of indifference, inattention, and withdrawal. In chronic cases where the paranoid symptom complex
is the leading clinical feature libidinal cathexis is invested in
fantasy objects of an erotic, supporting, or persecutory kind.

At the onset of these paranoid syndromes the cathexis of real
objects is retained alongside the pathologically enhanced

cathexis of the self. Different representations of the self, most of which previously existed as unconscious fantasies, enter consciousness as a consequence of their cathexis with libido. Omnipotent and omniscient ideas, alterations in sexual identity again based on unconscious fantasies, and other kinds of delusion relating to the self occur. Merging of self and object representations follows from the ease with which object cathexis gives way to self cathexis. This may result in a state where there is a fusion of the bodily boundaries of self and object. Concurrently with these changes there is a cathexis of delusional object representations.

These hypothesized internal changes are based on observations of the way in which patients relate to others at the onset of a psychosis. In contrast to the chronic patient whose interest in real objects is wholly dependent on need satisfactions, the early cases exhibit a combination of awareness and concern for real external objects, but they misidentify them with other object representations, real and fantasied.

Patients who have been able to make an object choice in reality, in contrast to those who have not, can, during the illness, still show interest and concern. Real external objects, for these patients, are not merely the means of need satisfaction. Sometimes they are regarded as serving the task of drive control. Such patients can sometimes respond to the offer of psychotherapy by virtue of their still having quantities of object libido which has maintained its noninstinctual quality.

Early cases of psychosis can also be differentiated according to the presence or absence of overt aggression, the intensity of the aggression, its quality and distribution. The appearance of aggression at the onset of a psychosis is usually due to anxiety arising from the delusional reality. Of greater significance is the destructiveness which is attributed to the persecutors. This destructive quality must be due to a qualitative change in the aggressive drives brought about by the psychosis.

Chronic patients who are withdrawn and negativistic have the greatest potential for violence. This may appear when the patient is disappointed or when attempts are made to strike up a relationship. This violent aggression is often closely tied to libidinal arousal, the hate substituting for the sexual affects.

There is also considerable evidence to indicate that this destructive aggressiveness, occurring at the onset of a psychosis, is associated with a course of illness which ends in deterioration. During a psychosis the patient either gives vent directly to sexual (genital) wishes or he is constantly assailed by persecutory influences, but the two tendencies do not appear together. These phenomena (direct instinct expression and persecutory delusions) indicate that there is an absence of stable repression. When there is direct libidinal drive expression, effective defense is in abeyance. When there are persecutory delusions, a defense has been established but one where externalization and projection are predominant.

Externalization of the unwanted drive derivatives does not prevent their emergence in consciousness, even though their origin is placed outside the self (attribution of responsibility). When projection is operative, it prevents the drive derivatives from reaching consciousness, as does repression. In withdrawn, negativistic patients the defense consists almost entirely of a primitive type of repression where there is a decathexis of the representations of material reality. In addition, there are alterations in the tone of the voluntary musculature which interfere with motility and the expression of drive. The unstable nature of these defenses is evidenced by the ease with which they are disrupted with the free expression of sexuality and aggression.

During the completion of a Profile attention is directed equally to the major areas of disturbance—drives, ego, and superego. It is then impossible to conclude that either the disorder by itself or the ego organization alone acts as the primary influence in symptom formation. Similarly, when a remission occurs, it cannot be attributed solely to a restoration of the libidinal distribution to its normal state. The changes in the ego and its defenses must be included in the formulation.

The evaluation of factors contributing to the appearance of the symptoms and the assessment of the possibilities of remission can also be achieved by an examination of the preillness personality. The schema makes provisions for this. In the majority of cases only limited quantities of libido reached the most advanced levels of psychosexual development in the preillness personality. In some cases, a stable heterosexual object choice was present. In other cases, real object choice was impermanent. When there was real functioning object relationship, constant or transitory, the choice of the object was made on the basis of narcissism. Last there are those patients whose object choice was confined to fantasy. In this group patients vary according to the stage at which the drives and the ego were arrested in their development.

In cases where a complete remission occurs recovery of the ego and redistribution of the libido have taken place simultaneously. When there is only a partial remission or when the patient is left with a defect, Profile studies suggest that while the ego has been largely reconstituted the libido has not returned to its optimal distribution. This is reflected in the inhibition of interest and initiative, lack of affect, and hypochondriasis. It is these phenomena which indicate that the libido still hypercathects the self at the expense of objects.

SYMPTOMATOLOGY AND CLASSIFICATION   Profile studies inevitably lead to considerations of classification of symptoms and syndromes. Descriptive psychiatry finds itself confronted with numerous clinical problems which classifications based on symptomatology find difficult to accommodate. Among these problems may be mentioned the combination of syndromes occurring during a single attack when elation of mood and psychomotor overactivity exist alongside persecutory delusions. Again there may be a transition from one syndrome to another. Psychomotor overactivity may be gradually replaced by a state characterized by withdrawal and cataleptic phenomena. A further difficulty for classification is presented by those patients in whom a different syndrome appears in two separate bouts of illness, for example, depressive phenomena in one attack and persecutory delusions in the next.

In transcending the purely descriptive approach the schema offers an alternative means of evaluating these clinical manifestations. The symptoms can be related to the state of the libidinal distribution, to conflicts, to defenses, and to regressions from the level achieved prior to the psychosis. When changes occur in symptoms and syndromes, Profiles illustrate the continuity between the phenomena and between one phase of illness and the next. If psychomotor overactivity is super-seded by withdrawal and negativism or elation by depression of mood and irritability, it can be seen that the new phenomena result from attempts to provide a defense organization which will restrain the expression of the drive derivatives. When a catatonic syndrome is suddenly replaced by the free outlet of sexuality and aggression, the change is due to the dissolution of the defenses which were effective until this time.

Familiarity with the schema and its concepts leads to a refinement of clinical description and to the possibility of a better differentiation of nosological entities. If patients who are given a diagnosis of paranoid schizophrenia are assessed from the standpoint of the existing defense organization, the delu-sional phenomena can be seen to vary with respect to the predominant defense mechanism. In some cases the defense achieves the aim of preventing affect and ideation from reach-ing consciousness. These patients complain of being regarded as sexually deviant; of being interfered with in different ways; of being subjected to unpleasant bodily experiences; and of being the objects of hate, jealousy, and envy. Here projection is the mainstay of the defense. In other cases, as was mentioned previously, the patient is aware of sexual and/or aggressive affects but attributes their stimulus to outside sources. Here the defense is that form of externalization known as attribution of responsibility. Projection plays no part in this.

Profiles completed on patients presenting these two different kinds of delusional experience at different stages of the illness suggest that major changes in the clinical picture, for better or worse, are more likely to occur in those whose principal de-fense is externalization rather than projection. Projection pro-vides the basis for a more stable clinical picture. While both externalization (attribution of responsibility) and projection alter the aim and the object of the libido, the circumstances necessary for their appearance differ. Projection will only act when the ego defect is minimal, while externalization does not require this precondition. The more extensive the regression affecting drives, ego, and superego, the more likely is exter-nalization to play a major role in defense. The fact of regres-sion always implies the possibility of the recovery of the ego and the return of the libido to reality without the necessity for the creation, through projection, of a delusional reality.

RESEARCH The schema has recently been used to compare and contrast psychotic states in children and adults. The study and treatment of children suffering from psychoses (Thomas et al., 1966) has revealed data which are almost identical with those found in psychoses occurring in early or middle life. The children who were treated presented nearly all the categories of symptomatology and abnormal behavior which are regarded by Creak et al. (1964) as characteristic of the schizophrenic syndrome in childhood. The adult patients who present phenomena similar to those encountered in the children are those in whom the psychosis has an acute onset (mania, reactive psychosis, etc.) with a relatively short course and those where the psychosis is in a state of chronicity (chronic schizophrenia) but is capable of sudden eruptions of affect, drive action, and delusion.

Similar manifestations are found in the spheres of interpersonal relationships and cognition. Like some adult patients, the children use the real external object (e.g., the therapist) as a source of need satisfaction or as a means of drive control. Again like adult patients, they show the same tendency to merge self and object representations. Speech and thinking disorders, perceptual and motility disturbances (catatonic signs, hyperkinesis) are also similar.

When the phenomena observed in the psychotic children are evaluated from the metapsychological standpoint, they can be understood in exactly the same way as is possible for the adult cases. The children are either unable to sustain object cathexis or have difficulty in doing so. The self is cathected at the expense of real objects whenever there is the slightest sign of endopsychic stress in the form of anxiety with a resulting movement toward the kind of primitive identification that is found in the adult patients. This merging process in its turn enhances the anxiety because of the fear of loss of identity (A. Freud, 1952).

A further similarity can be seen in the quality of the libidinal drives in the two categories of patients. In both the drives follow the primary process, seeking immediate outlets for their derivatives, with objects serving only as means of need satisfaction. It is the condensations and displacements which lead to the cognitive (thinking, perceiving, memory) disturbances and to the inappropriate affective expression.

We hope that the detailed comparison of Profiles of child and adult psychotic patients will throw some light on the *acquired,* as opposed to the *hereditary,* factors which predispose to these illnesses.

Summary

In this paper an attempt has been made to show how a Profile schema can be applied to the study of psychosis. Like the other schemata it represents the beginnings of efforts to present clinical data systematically and to assess their metapsychological significance. The reliability of the schema will ultimately depend on the experience, knowledge, and integrity of the psychoanalyst.

9

ANNA FREUD

The Nursery School of the Hampstead Child-Therapy Clinic

After working for a number of years with the middle-class children of the Clinic's neighborhood, our nursery school changed its orientation in 1967. From then onward it became our avowed purpose to serve the children of underprivileged and disadvantaged families and to inquire into the reasons for their frequent failure to adapt first to school, and later to the wider social community.

We assume that the developmental progress of any child depends on a number of favorable influences such as sufficient bodily care, membership in an intact and loving family, affection and support on a continuing basis, ongoing stimulation of his intellectual potentialities, and opportunity for identification with parents who themselves are healthy members of a community. Whenever in a child's upbringing one or more of these conditions are missing, the result is shown in arrests or deviations of development and/or failures in reaching the aims prescribed by the first social groups entered by the child.

Knowing full well that the above enumeration of the child's developmental needs is an ideal, rarely fulfilled in any class of society, we nevertheless feel convinced that social, financial, and racial pressures make it almost impossible for parents to meet their children's justified expectations.

We turned accordingly to the Social and Health Services of our Borough Council and informed them of the vacancies in our nursery school. They offered us for our final selection children in several categories whom they considered to be severely at risk.

Category A: Children of immigrant families where either both parents, or especially the mother, had not made adequate contact with their new cultural surroundings, and where either one or both parents had not yet mastered the English language. Such children usually grow up in close contact with their mothers, but isolated from the surrounding world and totally lacking in interest in or knowledge of it. Since their acquaintance with the English language is long delayed, they enter school tongue-tied and uncommunicative and often appear backward. They are unused to local food and customs and initially unable to enter into play with peers. Their deprivation of stimulation and of appropriate opportunities is usually exacerbated by the very poor housing conditions from which these families suffer.

Category B: Children of unmarried mothers or wives deserted by their husbands. These children are referred to us for various reasons. Some mothers work and relegate the children to unsuitable child-minders. Some live at home on National Assistance with the child as their only companion, isolated from all other influences. Some, to the detriment of the children, make them witnesses to their promiscuity and to scenes of violence.

Category C: English or Irish working-class families in poor circumstances. Children of this background are referred to us mainly for two reasons: (a) because of poor housing conditions forcing a number of people, adults as well as children, to share poor, inadequate, and unhealthy premises; (b) for reasons of mental illness, instability, or criminality on the part of one or both parents.

In the last seven years, 40 children, age 2-5 years, of all races and colors and creeds, coming from Ireland, England, Mediterranean countries, Africa, China, India, and the Caribbean, have attended our school.

Definition of the Task

We regard it as our nursery school's task to fill the gaps left for whatever reason in the parental care, irrespective of the fact whether these omissions are in the area of physical nurture, affectionate support, or mental stimulation. Clues to the individual child's particular deprivation are extracted from two sources. One is a detailed study of the child's behavior on entry into the nursery school, i.e., his ease or difficulty to separate from home; his trust or distrust in relation to the teachers or observers; his ability or inability to relate to peers; his enjoyment of or indifference to play material; his timidity or mastery of free movement on the playground; his reaction to praise and criticism; his ability or inability to comply with the nursery school routine. His attitudes in all these respects are assessed against the background of expectable age-adequateness. The second source is the teachers' knowledge of each child's home background. To avoid our parents' usual mistrust of "official interference" we try to handle this in a free and easy manner, trusting the first contacts made by the initial home visits, the daily meeting with parents at the beginning and end of a nursery day, and, above all, the mothers' unscheduled visits to the teachers, when, unexpectedly, confidences are poured out.

The data collected from both sources are carefully studied, collated, and presented to meetings of our Educational Unit. Such meetings occur weekly to discuss each child in turn. They are attended by the nursery school staff and their child-analytic advisor, by child therapy and medical students who function as observers, by the Clinic's pediatrician, and by representatives of the Clinic's analysts and child analysts, including the Clinic's Director. In discussion, the lines of action concerning each child are laid down and progress is assessed.

Procedures

PHYSICAL CARE IN THE NURSERY SCHOOL   In some instances, the physical neglect of a child is due to the mother's indifference to her offspring, or to her own bodily or mental illness or incapacity; in others, the reasons are purely external ones, such as the absence of proper washing or toilet facilities. Whatever the causes, such children appear in the nursery school unwashed, unkempt, and disheveled, and are entitled to receive from us what they are denied at home, namely, proper nourishment, cleanliness, help with toilet and eating habits, with blowing their noses, care for their hair, pretty clothes.

An example of this type was Jeannie, the youngest of a large family, quite beyond the mother's capacity to care for. At entry into the nursery school, Jeannie looked like the proverbial waif and stray, unkempt, smelly, clumsy, and unattractive to many children and adults for that reason. When she left the nursery to enter school, the same child impressed observers as a pretty, graceful, good-looking little girl, admired by many. How much Jeannie herself appreciated the care given to her was revealed in an incident when she watched the nursery school teacher sew up the holes in her small teddy bear and said thoughtfully: "He likes to be looked after by you, doesn't he?"

It is a well-known fact that good-looking, well-cared-for children not only have an increased self-respect but are also treated with greater respect and forbearance in school and by the adult community. Thus, a change such as the one experienced by Jeannie may well alter a child's whole outlook and experience of life.

THE NURSERY SCHOOL AS SUBSTITUTE PARENT   In the case of children who are unwanted and unloved at home, the nursery school provides an alternative home environment where they can feel appreciated and where their individual characteristics are acknowledged and respected. There is ample evidence that such children lose their sullenness and blossom out in the nursery school group. Their reciprocal positive relationship with the teacher causes noticeable spurts in all-round development.

For a variety of reasons, parents may be unable to support the child's adaptation to the outside world in a consistent manner. They are indulgent and punitive in turn, allowing freely at one moment what enrages them the next. As a result, such children enter nursery school confused in their moral standards and behavior. They profit greatly from an environment where rules are simple, firm, unshakable, and benevolent; in time such children become proud of their adherence to them.

THE NURSERY SCHOOL'S ROLE IN PROMOTING VERBAL-IZATION   The ability to express themselves verbally to the environment is delayed not only in those children who have to acquire English as their second language, but in all those whose parents are themselves not given to verbal communication, or not close enough to their children to stimulate their speech by intimate contact with them. The majority of the children who enter our nursery school do so with either absent or inadequate verbalization of their needs and wishes; instead they express their feelings by means of gestures, actions, temper tantrums, and other affective outbursts.

Our teachers accept it as their task to take over the parental role in this respect as well; to this end they use a maximum of carefully planned verbal interactions with the child. These range from the simple naming of objects in the room or in the picture book to sophisticated storytelling and to communication in the so-called "talking circle" where each child learns to report to teachers and fellow pupils on happenings at home, on personal opinions and experiences. In this manner, the children acquire language surprisingly fast and the result often far exceeds the parents' own capacity in this respect.

THE NURSERY SCHOOL AS A SOURCE OF STIMULATION AND EXPERIENCE All nursery schools accept it as their task to stimulate the child's mental capacities and skills. They achieve this by providing play materials such as soft toys, dolls, puzzles, constructive toys, pencils, paints, plasticene, and by offering swings, climbing frames, tricycles to promote motility. Necessary as these activities are, for the underprivileged child it is not sufficient if stimulation is restricted to the nursery school room itself, since this merely adds a second closed circle to the enclosure of the home surrounding. What such children are deprived of as a rule and what can be given to them by us is contact with the interesting and pleasurable aspects of the wider world such as visits to the park, the zoo, the local library, museums, participation in festive public events. Shopping expeditions are undertaken, not necessarily in groups, but with individual children who feel proud of being personally included in the adults' concerns and activities.

We have no doubt that varied experience of this kind is reflected in an expansion of the children's personalities. We also find it effective in reducing the difference between their intelligence test results and those attained by children who come from more fortunate home backgrounds.

THE NURSERY SCHOOL AS AN INFLUENCE ON FAMILY LIFE   It
is no surprise to anybody anymore that the parents' personalities and their daily actions exert a constant influence on
their children's growth and behavior. It is perhaps less well
known that any change in the children also has repercussions
on the happenings at home. We find that many of our children
take their newly acquired school behavior to their own homes
and that this leads to subtle changes in their parents' relationship to them, and occasionally to massive changes in the parents' whole outlook on their roles and tasks. It remains an open
question, of course, how much of this is accomplished by the
child himself, and how much has to be ascribed to the example
given by the nursery school teacher and the parents' growing
trust in her.

THE NURSERY SCHOOL AS PART OF THE HAMPSTEAD
CHILD-THERAPY COURSE AND CLINIC   Although the nursery
school functions as an independent unit, it profits at the same
time from being included in the organization of the Hampstead Child-Therapy Course and Clinic. There are instances
when school and home observations are not sufficient to highlight the reasons for a child's disturbed behavior. When this
happens, the Clinic's Diagnostic Service is at the disposal of the
nursery school. What this service can provide is a detailed
Developmental Profile of the child in question, i.e., a diagnostic
picture in which progress on all lines of development is assessed and deviations from the age-adequate norm are pointed
out. This makes it possible to locate pathological formations
wherever they occur in the child's personality and to scrutinize
them as to their origin.

When the child's failures or distortions of development are
so massive that they do not respond to the educational efforts
of the nursery school, the therapeutic service of the Clinic is
ready to take over and to provide child guidance, or mother
guidance, or child analytic treatment.

10

ROSE EDGCUMBE

The Border Between Therapy and Education

In this paper I shall consider certain differences in the aims and methods of therapy and education with particular reference to young children suffering from delays and distortions in the development of their ego functioning and object relationships.

There is no border at all between education and therapy as far as the usefulness of a psychoanalytic theory of childhood development is concerned. Both educator and therapist are aided in their handling of a child by the knowledge of normal developmental processes and stages as exemplified in Anna Freud's developmental Profile and concept of developmental lines (1965a). The border is to be found, rather, in the differing ways of using this understanding.

Education may be defined, in its widest sense, as the contribution of the environment to the development and maturation of the individual's personality, capacities, skills, and talents. In this sense, the first and most important educators are the child's parents. In a narrower sense, and the one with which I am mainly concerned in this paper, education is the contribution made by the child's teachers to his development, especially in the areas of learning and socialization. Education is essentially directed toward strengthening and enlarging the ego: it seeks, by means of external stimulation, guidance, and example, to tame drive behavior; to divert drive energy into play, learning, and work activities; to promote adaptive defenses; to encourage sublimation of drive impulses and wishes via the

From the Educational Unit.

133

development of interests, skills, and talents; to aid the growth of independence from primary objects in thinking and behavior; and to establish a wide variety of mature relationships through the enjoyment of interaction and cooperation with peers and teachers. All this is done by means of an appeal to the child's predominantly conscious and rational interests, wishes, and standards; and it is a part of normal upbringing.

Therapy, in contrast, is a process which is brought into play only when a child's development is seriously disturbed. The specific form of therapy I have in mind is, of course, child psychoanalysis, primarily intended for the treatment of a specific type of disturbance: childhood neurosis. Analysis directs the child's attention inward, to the exploration of his internal psychic situation, seeking by means of interpretation to bring into consciousness areas of unconscious conflict, sometimes weakening defenses in its efforts to put the child in touch with his drive impulses, wishes, and fantasies.

Thus at times the inward-looking process of analysis may run counter to the outward-oriented process of education, at any rate until therapy has enabled the child's ego to arrive at better adapted compromises between the demands of id, superego, and external world, thus freeing the child's capacity to benefit from educational opportunities.

The teacher of the normal child and the therapist of the neurotic child both rely on the child's having a relatively well-functioning ego and a good enough capacity for object relationships to make use of the experiences offered to him within a relationship. But teacher and therapist make different uses of these capacities in the child.

The teacher offers himself, his ideals, interests, and standards as models with which the child can identify; and he seeks to gain the child's trust, affection, and respect. Initially, this positive relationship fosters in the child the development of a wish to please the teacher, to gain his admiration and approval; the teacher can use this wish to make constructive play, learning, and work, both alone and in cooperation with other children, pleasurable and rewarding activities for the child. Subsequently the child moves toward autonomy in these areas of functioning; and success in them becomes an internalized source of self-esteem.

The therapist uses the neurotic child's capacities for relationships and ego functioning in two ways. Child and therapist must form a therapeutic alliance in which both can work toward understanding the child's internalized conflicts, in spite of the temporary loss of self-esteem and increase of anxiety, guilt, and shame this process may arouse in the child. And an important part of the analytic process is the child's transference onto the therapist of negative as well as positive aspects of his relationships: for example, he is hostile as well as affectionate, seeks to defy as well as to please, provokes blame and punishment as well as praise and reward.

Teacher and therapist alike are faced with difficulties when, for whatever reasons, the child is unable to form sufficiently mature or stable relationships and when his ego functioning is not adequate to cope adaptively with the demands made on him by the educational or therapeutic process. In these circumstances, the teacher may resort to techniques which may broadly be described as therapeutic, while the therapist may use techniques which are, in the widest sense, educative. Both are trying to remedy delays or distortions in the child's personality development. This partial overlapping of techniques can sometimes lead to a blurring of the distinction between education and therapy. The border between the two can perhaps best be traced by reference to the aims of each, as well as to the nature and origins of the disturbances which determine the method of handling most appropriate for a particular problem. To illustrate this, I would like to discuss some of the under-fives who attend the Hampstead Clinic Nursery School, run by Mrs. Friedmann.

Our nursery school is intended for normal children, but, like any school, it has always found it necessary to cope with a small proportion of disturbed children. About six years ago we switched from admitting mainly middle-class children from the immediate neighborhood to taking mainly children from poorer districts who were thought by their local medical and social welfare workers to be especially deprived or disadvantaged because of poor socioeconomic status, family difficulties, or mental ill-health in the parents. This has somewhat increased the proportion of children in the nursery school who are found to be suffering from delayed or distorted development in object relationships and ego functioning.

This group of children is of special interest to us because of the diagnostic problems they pose, and the concomitant difficulties in selecting the form of special help most appropriate to each. In addition, there are certain practical difficulties to be overcome which are common to most schools. First, since the children are not referred for treatment, we do not start out with diagnostic interviews, and we have only limited information on the child's personal and social history. Most of our knowledge of the child's difficulties is therefore gained from observation of the child in the nursery school. Second, many of the parents of these children are unaware of their child's disturbance; when they are aware of it, they may be unable or unwilling to support psychoanalytic treatment because of their anxieties, depression, or preoccupation with other problems. But they usually welcome any attention the child receives within the normal school setting.

Largely because of these practical difficulties we tend, in our attempts at working with a disturbed child, to start by experimenting with various ways of special handling within the nursery school setting, only later adding individual help outside the school. Consequently there is an ongoing interaction between the processes of assessment and attempted treatment.

Initially we have to decide between three possible general assessments. First, the behavior we see may simply be a sign of normal, phase-adequate developmental immaturity which the child will outgrow in his own time. Second, it may be a transitory developmental disturbance, that is, a phase-adequate conflict or a temporary reaction to some environmental event which the child will overcome with no special help other than ordinary sympathetic handling. Third, it may be a potentially permanent disturbance which will persist or deteriorate unless the child receives special help. It is particularly difficult to decide between these three possibilities in the case of young

children, and ours are sometimes as young as 2½ years. Often
one can only wait and see.

Christine, for example, started nursery school early, at the
age of 2 years and 9 months, as an emergency measure because
her mother was in the hospital. She was an intelligent, lively,
inquisitive toddler who darted about, exploring and often
upsetting everything. She followed the teachers around, getting
under their feet, demanding instant satisfaction of her desires
in a piercing voice. She made sporadic disruptive forays into
the games and activities of other children, not wanting to be
left out, but unable to understand what was going on or join in
cooperatively. Her squeaks of "Me, too!" became a familiar
sound in the school. Her behavior was sympathetically tolerated by the other children as well as by the adults because of
her young age and the current separation from her mother.

Christine was the youngest of six, her siblings ranging in age
from 7 to 22 years. Her brother had been a star pupil in the
nursery school, and we thought her working-class family to be
well-functioning and happy. Outside nursery hours she was
being looked after at home by her father and older sister. We
confidently expected her to surmount the separation from her
mother and to settle down as she reached the normal entry age
of 3.

During the following year, however, her functioning remained negatively focused on ensuring that she was not ignored by the teachers, not excluded from any activities, that
nobody got anything more or better than she did. Yet, as soon
as she was accepted into a group, allowed to join in an activity,
or given what she wanted, she lost interest. She was often sad,
listless, or tearful.

Since our head teacher has one, and sometimes two, assis-
tants for about 12 children, a child like Christine can be given a
great deal of individual attention; but Christine could not really
enjoy being alone with one teacher. She was constantly on the
alert in case she was missing something else. The teacher could
not stimulate Christine's interest in games and activities, either
for the sake of the pleasure they gave her, or for the sake of
getting the adult's praise for her skills and achievements. Nor

could she enjoy the more regressed relationship she often seemed to want: she could not, for example, settle comfortably on an adult's lap. No amount of attention and interest seemed to reassure Christine that she was wanted and liked, no amount of praise and admiration could raise her abysmally low self-esteem. The behavior which had been acceptable and even charming in a toddler was intrusive, irritating, and frustrating in a 4-year-old, so that Christine was beginning to provoke the very dislike and rejection she so much feared; and we learned that this was so at home as well as in the nursery school. The negative aspects of her relationships and the reasons for her low self-esteem had to be understood, and the conflicts which were preventing her development out of the ambivalently clinging and tormenting toddler type of relationship had to be resolved before she could progress. Only analysis could fulfill these requirements.

Christine illustrates one of the questions we have to answer when deciding between remedial educational techniques and psychotherapy: can the child establish a positive relationship with the teacher that is strong enough to exclude the problems which bedevil other relationships? Christine could not: she transferred onto her teachers both her mistrust of her primary objects and her ambivalence to them; and onto her peers she transferred her envy and jealousy of her siblings.

Other children can establish a positive relationship with a teacher in spite of their difficulties. This may be because they manage to circumvent the internalized conflicts which affect their relationships to primary objects: we are all familiar with the child who is angelic in school and a demon at home. Or the teacher may be able to avoid arousing the fears or entering into the external conflicts the child has with primary objects, and give the child a new experience of relationships.

An example of this was Matthew, the youngest child of a poor family living in slum conditions. His mother was of average intelligence, but his father and three older siblings were all subnormal. Mrs. Friedmann had met Matthew during her visits to a neighboring nursery school family, and as a baby and toddler he had seemed friendly and lively, more intelligent than the rest of the family. Then his mother went out to work and he was placed with a child minder during the day. When he joined the nursery school at 2 years 9 months his mother warned us that we would hear "terrible language." But we heard almost nothing, since he spoke little to adults, although he talked to other children. In general he seemed dull and inert, often vacant, obediently falling in with nursery routine, but showing little spontaneous interest in activities; he seemed quite frightened of the teachers.

We speculated whether he was, after all, a child of low intelligence, bewildered by the level of activities in the nursery school; whether the separation from his mother had disrupted his relationships and general development; or whether he had been intimidated or ill-treated by his parents or the woman who had minded him.

The teachers made special efforts to allay Matthew's fear of them, approaching him gently and carefully, trying to find games he could enjoy and things he could talk about. Matthew in fact selected from what was offered the forms of remedial education he needed, and two things seem to have been particularly helpful.

One was the availability of men among our observers, drawn from students and visitors, who regularly spend time in the nursery school. Being less afraid of men than of women, Matthew began approaching male observers, at first engaging them in boisterous physical games such as he enjoyed with his father, and bossing them around. These contacts could then be extended to more varied and sophisticated games, activities, and outings, all of which he enjoyed.

Simultaneously, everyone was making special efforts to encourage Matthew to speak. We had observed that he often seemed to be muttering under his breath, and tried to get close enough to hear. The first things we heard were eminently sensible. For example, while passively allowing the teacher to change his shoes, he was heard to mutter, "Them are not my shoes"—and he was right.

For some time, in spite of encouragement, Matthew remained apparently afraid to speak his thoughts aloud to adults. Nor would he join in the children's "talking circle" with the teacher; until one day he overheard a discussion about accidents. This captured his attention and provoked him into telling a long fantasy about his brother having an accident, being dead and going to the hospital. This was the beginning of a series of fantasies about accidents, injuries, and deaths, and with this Matthew began to come to life: he became increasingly communicative, adventurous, and boisterous; eventually he was well able to master all available activities in the school, and to make good relationships with the women teachers.

We speculated that inhibition of aggressive wishes or an attempt to control fears of being hurt had been the cause of his previous dullness and inertia; and we wondered whether his ego was strong enough to control his newly emerging impulses; also whether there would prove to be conflicts requiring psychotherapy. But being allowed to tell his fantasies and discuss them with adults on a reality level was all that Matthew needed; and there was no inappropriate discharge into action apart from a brief episode of rough and slightly sadistic handling of the school's hamsters.

It seemed that Matthew had largely been suffering from lack of intellectual stimulation and opportunities for imaginative talk and play at home. If he had been intimidated or unduly restricted by adults, he had not yet internalized the restriction: friendly and sympathetic adults could still elicit a different response. His intelligence proved to be above average, and he settled well in primary school at age 5. We felt that in Matthew's case the teachers and observers had been able to supply the stimulation of intellectual functioning and the ego support in dealing with fears and impulses that were missing in his relationships at home, and this had been sufficient to promote normal development.

We have found this to be true for other children whose developmental delays in ego functioning and object relationships were due to the parents' inability to provide adequate support and stimulation. But the age of the child on entry into the nursery school is one important factor in determining how effectively educational measures can supplement and counteract the child's experience at home. This is why we have begun admitting some children before the usual age of 3.

This point is illustrated by two boys from another family, the Rileys, who also lived in overcrowded slum conditions, but parents and children had average intelligence. Of the six children, three were already in state schools, where their difficulties were such that they were thought to be educationally subnormal. The fourth child, Keith, entered our nursery school at age 4. Unlike Matthew, Keith was an outgoing, friendly urchin, likable, but almost unmanageable. He threw himself into activities with great gusto, but without control, getting immense enjoyment but upsetting everyone else in the process. He was easily discouraged in activities which proved at all difficult; his vocabulary was limited and his indistinct speech was used mainly for bellowing his wishes at maximum volume; he could not wait his turn or share toys; he bashed every child who got in his way or had something he wanted; and he usually reacted to frustration with major tantrums (followed by collapse into silent misery) which have become a legend in the recent history of the nursery school. His bowel and bladder control were precarious; he had a runny nose; and he was often grubby and smelly.

We felt daunted by the tasks which had to be accomplished in one year before this disorganized child entered primary school, particularly as we feared that his impulsiveness and low frustration tolerance might already be an established part of his character structure. Fortunately, although Keith's mode of relating was immature, his capacity for relationships was strong and he approached objects with trust and good expectations. His wish to be loved and admired by the teachers made him cooperate with their efforts, which were essentially exaggerations of normal teaching techniques: lavish praise and rewards for achievements and good behavior, very stern reprimands and punishments for bad behavior; frequent, careful explanations of what was expected of him and why his behavior was acceptable or not; individual help in mastering games and tasks to enable him to catch up with other children. Perhaps the only unusual technique was the introduction of regular bathing and hair-washing sessions (in addition to toilet training and nose wiping) to help promote pride in the appearance of his body and the control of its functions.

We felt that we had barely managed to get Keith ready for entry to primary school in spite of delaying his entry for an extra three months. His achievements were still precarious, even though he managed to fit into his class with only occasional fights and tantrums and to keep up with the work. Our experience with Keith made us take in his younger brother Paul earlier, at the age of 2½. Paul and Keith were very similar in personality and development and a shudder went round the staff meeting the day Mrs. Friedmann reported: "Paul has tantrums in the true Keith style." However, being younger, Paul's difficulties were less entrenched than Keith's had been and, of course, we had a longer period of time to work with him; so that when the time came for Paul to move on to primary school we were more confident that he would do well.

The Riley family also provides a cautionary example of the way in which different children in the same environment may be quite differently affected. In between Keith and Paul was a girl, Joan, who entered nursery school at age 3, simultaneously with Keith. Joan showed delayed development in object relationships and disorganized ego functioning similar to her brothers, but she was more passive, less unruly, and prone to whining rather than tantrums. Her passivity proved to be a sign that she lacked her brothers' active, albeit disorganized, push toward development and mastery. Her interests seemed fleeting and easily lost; no lasting desires or aims could be elicited; wishes for admiration and praise could not be mobilized; she continued to look, and apparently to feel, neglected and unlovable; she seemed unable to compete for attention or even to hang on to her own possessions. Her only constant pleasure was to sit on a lap, kissing and cuddling in infantile fashion; but she was indiscriminate, seeking out any unoccupied adult, even a stranger.

Joan's inability to form an emotional attachment to a particular adult handicapped the teachers in their attempts to work with her. By the time she was 4 it was clear that she needed the peace and quiet of a period of time alone with one adult away from the distractions of group life, but it was unclear what form this individual help should take since the nature of her disturbance was uncertain.

The therapist's first task with Joan was simply to follow, verbalize, and gratify whatever demands and needs could be discerned in an attempt to find a pattern in them. This kind of gratification was neither analytic nor educative, but it was an essential first step to meeting the child on her own level in order to examine her functioning with an analyst's eye. It encouraged Joan's positive emotional attachment to the therapist, on the basis of which Joan could then move on to demand that her therapist do other things besides holding and caring for her. What became clear during this phase of treatment was that, although Joan had many disparate wishes on the drive side and many interests on the ego side, she could initiate nothing herself, but simply wanted things provided or done for her.

It was next possible to combine educational techniques of gradually limiting gratification and encouraging Joan to try things for herself with analytic exploration of her reactions to this increasing pressure from her therapist. Anger, sadness, feelings of frustration and even guilt and shame began to emerge; and therapist and child could explore why Joan felt so frightened of the object's refusal to comply with her wishes, why she dare not become more independent in trying things out for herself, and why she so easily felt defeated and worthless when she could not immediately succeed at an attempted activity. The therapist could begin to distinguish defensive regressions and confusions from developmental delays and environmentally produced confusion.

As the analytic delineation of Joan's chaotic inner world proceeded, the elements could be put together into recognizable conflicts and defenses and their effect on her development could be traced. For example, one of Joan's own contributions to the impoverishment of her self representation proved to have been the excessive use of primitive defense mechanisms of externalization and projection: Joan disowned any aspect of herself which she disliked and which could arouse shame, anxiety, or guilt. One defensive element in her passivity proved to be the need to shift responsibiltiy for approving and gratifying her wishes onto the object.

Joan's consistent disowning of wishes and her renunciation

of aspirations had rendered her teachers powerless to mobilize active and progressive forces in her. Her treatment enabled her to accept these wishes and aspirations as part of herself and to seek more adaptive ways of handling them. It was an important moment when Joan's sense of identity and her growing awareness that she might be able to feel good about herself reached a point where she could formulate the question to her therapist: "How do I be proud of myself?"

As Joan's analysis proceeded, the functions of her therapist and teachers could be gradually separated, so that her therapist could concentrate on the clarification and interpretation of Joan's conflicting wishes, fears, and feelings about herself, while her teachers now could effectively take over the more direct stimulation and support of progressive developmental moves.

In the cases reported so far we had at least passive support from parents who were pleased by the changes in their children; and the parental contribution to their children's disturbance had mainly taken the form of inadequacies or omissions in their handling. The problems are different, of course, where parents actively refuse or undermine the help offered to the children, or where parental pathology is such that even if they accept help we know that we can do little to counteract the ongoing malign influence of the parents.

Robert, for example, had lived alone in a one-room flat with his mother since the age of 6 months when his parents were divorced. Mrs. H. was a borderline psychotic woman who reacted to Robert on the basis of her own needs, not his, and expected his feelings to coincide with hers. She identified Robert with his father, whom she saw as a dishonest, sexually promiscuous and murderous psychopath. Her view of her husband was probably as distorted by her own projections as was her view of Robert. Her terror that Robert would become antisocial or a criminal like his father made her berate him constantly for being "bad"—which meant failing to comply instantly with her wishes. If anyone else criticized Robert, she defended her son with tigresslike ferocity, blaming the trouble on other badly brought-up children, or on antagonistic adults.

She seemed incapable of speaking in anything other than a loud, hoarse voice; she sometimes lost her temper and hit Robert quite viciously, or threatened to send him away. At the same time she was sexually seductive, allowing him to see her undressed, to share her bed, and encouraging much kissing and cuddling. She denied, however, that he was ever sexually excited or curious in spite of clear evidence to the contrary. In between times she often smothered him with inappropriate caring.

Robert entered the nursery school at age 3½. He was intellectually precocious, especially in speech, which had an oddly adult quality; ego control over drives and affects was poor; he was restless, tense, distractible, easily excitable; he took pleasure in teasing and interfering with other children and often threatened and attacked them so fiercely that they were frightened and had to be protected from him; and he was himself subject to fits of screaming panic for no obvious reasons. Although somewhat reassured by the consistency and predictability of the teachers, he remained rather mistrustful and distant, which was not surprising in view of his mother's inconsistent, confusing, and often frightening behavior and her almost complete inability to empathize with his feelings or meet his needs.

Mrs. H. accepted psychotherapy for Robert and guidance for herself, though little could be done in interviews with her except to channel some of her anxiety, hostility, and seductiveness away from Robert. There was a constant danger that she would interrupt Robert's treatment because of her fear that he might be labeled a psychiatric case. However, his therapist was able to work with Robert to some extent on his fears of punishment and rejection arising from his conflicts over aggressive and sadistic sexual impulses and to distinguish the neurotic anxiety resulting from projection of these impulses from realistic anxiety about his mother's behavior. One important area of analysis centered on his various identifications, including, first, those with various aspects of his crazy mother—a normal process, but using an abnormal object; second, a defensive identification with the aggressor (his mother as well as other objects onto whom he had projected his own impulses); third, an identification with his mother's view of him as murderous and dangerous.

Robert's aggressiveness and panic in the nursery school diminished and, though his relationships remained distant, he seemed able to gain pleasure and relief from absorption in intellectual pursuits. His primary school found him slightly difficult, but he was less of a problem to them than his mother. Since his treatment finished, at age 6, the sadomasochistic tie with his mother seems to have intensified again. We sometimes meet them in the street walking along with arms around each other, but with expressions of suppressed fury.

In the examples I have given, I have described some of the methods we have tried for helping young children with disturbances in the development of their object relationships and ego functioning. Some of them, of course, have difficulties in other areas as well; but I have selected these areas because problems in them are usually closely related developmentally and because they are the areas in which the therapeutic efforts of teachers and child analysts meet and overlap.

I have indicated that where a child's ability to profit from educational experience is being interfered with by internalized conflicts, or by distortions in his modes of relating and functioning of a kind which preclude his making a predominantly positive and trusting relationship to his teacher, then individual psychotherapy is required. Such children require analytic exploration and interpretation of their internal world, in a one-to-one relationship, away from the distractions of the school group. In some cases the therapist may have to borrow more directly educational techniques, at least in the initial stages of treatment, in order to boost a child's functioning, mode of relating, and self-esteem to a point where the demands of analysis proper can be tolerated and its insights used effectively. But it would not be appropriate to attempt analytic work within the school itself, because of the disruption to group life which can arise from enactment of conflicts, transference of negative features of relationships, and the proliferation of fantasies.

Remedial work within the school setting seems more appropriate than analysis for children whose difficulties are not the product of conflict or of malign environmental influences on their mode of relating and identifications, but which result mainly from inadequacies or omissions in their earlier relationships and upbringing in their home environment. Even though these children's modes of relating may be immature, provided they still have the basic capacity to form a positive relationship, skilled and sensitive teachers can use extensions and modifications of normal educational methods to help these children catch up in their development. For many children, nursery school attendence can itself be, in a broad sense, a therapeutic experience, because of the stability and predictability of the setting and the consistency and reliability of the staff.

Finally, at the risk of saying what everyone knows already, I would like to stress again one technique which is as important for the teacher as for the therapist when working with children such as I have described: that is the use of verbalization of the child's feelings, wishes, reactions, and experiences in general. Whether the aim is to help the child get the most out of what the environment has to offer, or whether it is to help him understand his inner world, verbalization is the main tool in clarifying and making sense of experiences for the child, in helping him to think rather than act, and in establishing two-way communication with other people.

11

JOSEPH SANDLER

Sexual Fantasies and Sexual Theories in Childhood

In the early 1960s the Hampstead Index Research group began a study of children's sexual fantasies and theories. This study was initiated as a result of the difficulties which therapists and Index workers had found in suitably defining and classifying material which might be called "fantasy," derived from psychoanalytic treatment of children at the Clinic. We had known from past experience with the Index (Sandler, 1962) that such difficulties of categorization and classification pointed to ambiguities and other problems in regard to the definition of the terms and concepts used.

I

As part of an intensive study of the concepts of fantasy and unconscious fantasy, the following observations were made (Sandler and Nagera, 1963):

1. In addition to conscious daydreams reported by the child, therapists tended to include, under the heading of "fantasy," many other types of verbal reports made by the child if these were at all distorted by the child's own inner wishes, thoughts, and past experiences. Theories which were "childish" (but perhaps age-appropriate) as well as transference distortions and speculations about the therapist tended to be included.

2. Material was often labeled "fantasy" when it referred to nonverbal expressions such as dramatization and painting. In-

From the Index Research Group.

149

deed, almost every derivative of the patient's unconscious mental life tended, at times, to be classified as "fantasy."

3. The recorded fantasy often contained a mixture of the patient's material and the therapist's interpretation of that material.

4. In the recorded fantasies no clear differentiation seemed to be made between the role of instinctual wishes, affects, repressed memories, preconscious thoughts, and repressed earlier fantasies which reappeared in distorted form.

5. When an attempt was made to classify "fantasy" material under the heading of "latent fantasy themes," an endless variety of headings relating to drives, unconscious content, pregenital fixations, affects, and defenses emerged.

6. It appeared to be impossible to make a clear differentiation between fantasies and theories, especially sexual fantasies and sexual theories.

As a first step, a systematic study of Freud's views on fantasy was made. The outcome of this is summarized below.

Freud used the term "fantasy" in a number of ways, including both conscious daydreams and their unconscious counterparts. However, a theory of fantasy does emerge in Freud's work, largely developed before the introduction of the structural theory in 1923. *Conscious daydream fantasies* can be considered to be wish-fulfilling products of the imagination, which are known not to be real. When they acquire belief, they are no longer daydreams but rather are delusions, hallucinations, or dreams (during the dreaming state). Daydream fantasies have two sets of determinants, one conscious, the other unconscious. The daydream represents a compromise between the two. Daydream fantasying begins during children's play, and is a split-off type of thought activity in which dependence on real objects has been abandoned.

Daydream fantasies function to gratify repressed and secret wishes and to protect the ego from anxiety arising from undischarged instinctual tension. The wish fulfillments of fantasy compensate for the insufficient gratification provided by reality. They also serve to exonerate the person from feelings of guilt by "embellishing" the facts. In this connection, Freud referred to fantasies as "defensive structures" (Letter No. 61 to Fliess).

Fantasies can be regarded as a substitute for play when the need for secrecy arises. The production of daydreams helps the child to become independent of the external world by finding "internal " satisfaction. Sexual fantasies have a direct developmental link with masturbation, and allow a gratification of the child's unconscious sexual wishes, as well as wishes from the sphere of object love.

Freud connected the emergence of daydream fantasy in the child with the development of the reality principle. As the reality principle develops, fantasy becomes increasingly "split off" from other forms of thinking. Fantasy functions in this context as a compensation for abandoned forms of gratification. The imagination is, according to Freud (1911), exempted from the demands of reality testing.

Daydream fantasies are, like dreams, built up out of previous impressions. Indeed, they share many of their properties with nocturnal dreams. Both are wish fulfillments, based largely on infantile impressions, and both benefit by some relaxation of the censorship. Both combine elements of the past with present-day impressions.

Freud (1908a) pointed out that the two main groups of wishes concerned in daydreams are the ambitious and the erotic. The daydream allows the link with the real object to be maintained, even though it may be diminished in actual life. The daydream involves some *current* impression which arouses a major wish. It recalls memories of satisfying *past* experiences and creates a *future* situation which is the wish fulfillment.

All the above relates to the conscious daydream, but Freud had a great deal to say about unconscious fantasies. Mental content which is *descriptively* unconscious may belong to the *system* Unconscious or to the Preconscious. Only certain contents of the Preconscious are available to consciousness, as preconscious material may itself be subject to censorship and be prevented from acquiring the property of consciousness. (The second censorship, between the Preconscious and the Conscious was postulated by Freud in 1915.)

It follows that when Freud spoke of unconscious fantasies he referred both to fantasies in the system Unconscious and fantasies in the Preconscious. Fantasies in the Unconscious consist of memories of past wish-fulfilling fantasies which had subsequently been repressed and, being in the Unconscious, were subject to primary process functioning. Fantasies in the Preconscious, while *descriptively* unconscious, are subject to secondary process thinking, and may, to some extent, represent wish fulfillments which never acquire the property of consciousness.

The sources of unconscious fantasy may be summarized as follows (Sandler and Nagera, 1963):

1. Repressed memories and daydreams.
2. Fantasies which have been subjected to elaboration in the system *Ucs.* according to primary process laws.
3. Daydream derivatives of unconscious fantasies which have gained consciousness in a new form and which have again been repressed.
4. Derivatives of unconscious [wishes and] fantasies which have been elaborated in the system *Pcs,* but which have been repressed into the system Unconscious before reaching consciousness [p. 172].

Freud also pointed out that both conscious and preconscious daydreams can be tolerated as long as their level of intensity is not too great. If this level increases above a certain point, conflict may occur, with subsequent repression of the daydream into the system Unconscious. The instinctual wish, previously satisfied in the fantasy, may now have to find an outlet by means of a different type of derivative. If a satisfactory alternative derivative is not found, neurotic symptoms may develop.

Unconscious fantasies are regarded as possessing *psychic reality* in contrast to material reality.[1] They were seen by Freud as

---

[1] This raises a problem of definition, because we may legitimately ask whether the loss of the knowledge of "unreality" attached to unconscious thoughts still enables us to call some of these thoughts fantasies. It would appear that unconscious fantasies, to the degree to which they possess psychic reality, might perhaps more appropriately be regarded as "unconscious delusions," although this in turn raises further problems of definition and other complications.

playing a crucial part in determining the form and content of later daydreams. However, unconscious fantasies may also enter into the formation of types of derivatives other than fantasy. For example, they play an important part in the formation of neurotic and psychotic symptoms.

It is of some interest that Freud emphasized that a fantasy might be tolerated as a daydream, with the knowledge that it is a daydream, but if it comes too close to reality, it may then be subjected to repression.

Once a fantasy has been repressed into the system Unconscious, it no longer functions as a wish fulfillment as it did originally, but now becomes the content of an *unsatisfied wish*. The degree to which repressed fantasy material is cathected by the instinctual drive represents the degree to which there is a desire to reexperience it. Work analogous to the dreamwork may then have to take place in order to allow the disguised fulfillment of the particular instinctual wish.

It follows that a whole range of derivatives, including dreams, daydreams, works of art, other creative productions, symptoms and the like, may represent the concealed satisfaction of instinctual wishes which have as their content not only memories of past satisfactions, but also memories of wish-fulfilling daydreams.

At this point the essential points in Freud's writings on fantasy can be summed up:

1. Conscious fantasying or daydreaming is a reaction to frustrating external reality. It implies the creation of a wish-fulfilling situation in the imagination, thereby bringing about a temporary lessening of instinctual tension. Reality testing is discarded, but the ego nevertheless remains aware that the imaginative construction is not reality, without this knowledge interfering with the gratification thus achieved. Conscious fantasy differs from hallucinatory wish fulfillment in that the daydream is not normally confused with reality, whereas the hallucinatory gratification cannot be distinguished from reality.

2. Fantasies which are *descriptively* unconscious can be divided into two main classes: (i) those which are formed in the system Preconscious, and which parallel the formation of con-

scious daydreams, except that they do not possess the quality of consciousness; and (ii) those which are relegated by repression to the system Unconscious. To the repressed daydreams in the system Unconscious we must add the proliferated derivatives of fantasies and memories which have been formed according to the laws of the primary process, as well as derivatives which have reached the systems Preconscious and Conscious, subjected to secondary process elaboration and then repressed. For the sake of completeness, we can add the hypothetical primal or inherited fantasies.[2]

3. Once a conscious or preconscious fantasy has been repressed into the system Unconscious, it functions exactly like a *memory of instinctual satisfaction* and can provide the ideational content of the instinctual wishes. Fantasies in the system Unconscious—perhaps we can say "unconscious fantasies proper"—are *not* wish fulfillments, but are *now the ideational content of instinctual wishes.* They deserve the name of fantasy only inasmuch as they are derived from the content of conscious or preconscious fantasies. Fantasies belonging to the system Unconscious and those in the system Preconscious and Conscious may be similar in their ideational content. They can be contrasted in the descriptive, dynamic, and topographical senses.

4. Unconscious fantasies can find expression in new conscious and preconscious daydreams; but they can also find expression and gratification in any one of a large number of other forms, none of which necessarily qualifies for the designation "fantasy."

Some of the formulations made by Freud in regard to nocturnal dreams can also be extended to fantasies. The consideration of anxiety dreams, punishment dreams, and dreams showing the fulfillment of masochistic trends, in the context of wish fulfillment, allows us to extend the same considerations in regard to the theory of dreams to the theory of fantasy and to the understanding of anxiety fantasies, punishment fantasies, and masochistic fantasies.

From the structural point of view, it is not difficult to allocate those unconscious fantasies which were previously located in

---

[2] A topic not discussed in this paper.

the system Unconscious to the *id*. Fantasies in the system Preconscious can be regarded as being located in the unconscious part of the *ego*. We found it necessary in the Index research group to distinguish between the capacity of the ego to organize mental content, using a degree of secondary process functioning, and the *organized form* imposed on the mental content which is an outcome of the ego's work. Once formed by the ego, fantasy content which has been repressed, and then becomes the content of an instinctual wish in the id, may retain all or part of the organized qualities which have been imposed on it. This is, of course, true not only of fantasies, but also for the memories arising from reality perception. The process of *fantasying* can be regarded as an ego function, producing organized, wish-fulfilling, imaginative content, which may or may not become conscious. It involves a temporary laying aside of reality, although elements of reality can be utilized in the creation of the fantasy. Once formed by the ego, the fantasy content, which may show a high degree of organization and symbolization, can be repressed and be subject to primary process functioning alone. The difference between fantasy thinking and reality-orientated thinking was regarded as lying precisely in the fact that in fantasy the demands of reality are relatively ignored. The fantasy involves the creation of an alternative and satisfying "reality," which is, however, known not to be "real." But it is necessary to point out that many thoughts occupy an intermediate position between fantasy and reality-oriented thoughts, the two cases representing the extreme ends of a continuum.

It was felt that the following considerations would have to be taken into account in any consideration of fantasy (Sandler and Nagera, 1963):

1. As ideational contents may originate from a number of sources, it would appear to be inappropriate to use the term "fantasying" for the primary process elaboration of these contents into the ideational content of instinctual wishes. It is only when the ego participates in the organization of content into wish-fulfilling imaginative products that we should speak of fantasying or fantasy formation.

2. Fantasying as an ego function results in organized,

wish-fulfilling, imaginative content, which may or may not be consciously perceived. The fantasy may then be a derivative, a compromise constructed by the ego between the instinctual wish and the demands of the superego. Reality knowledge may be suspended in the formation of this derivative, or it may be utilized and may influence the fantasy to a high degree. The fantasy content may be repressed soon after it has been created, or defended against in other ways.

3. The fantasy is only one of many derivatives which the ego can construct.

4. Some fantasies represent wish fulfillments when the wish in question arises neither from the id, nor from the superego, but from the ego itself.

5. In normal mental functioning repressed content may be derived from memory images of all sorts, including those of wish-fulfilling fantasies, "real" experiences, dreams, reality-orientated thoughts. On the other hand, derivatives of the repressed (indicating a "return of the repressed") may be expressed in perceptual images, wishes, acts, reality-orientated thinking, dreams, play, free associations, screen memories, distorted recollections of the past, manifest transference content, symptoms, delusions, scientific theories, hypnagogic phenomena, artistic and literary creations as well as daydream fantasies.

In all of this a distinction has to be made between "id-cathected content," subject to primary process alone, forming the content of instinctual wishes, on the one hand, and "ego-modified content," on the other. Because repressed id-cathected content is not normally permitted direct and undisguised discharge, it can achieve this only through the formation of derivatives. It was assumed that in order to circumvent the censorship, some degree of modification and organization of the purely instinctually cathected content must occur before the ego can permit the derivative to have access to consciousness and motility.

In these processes there is a constant "back and forth" movement, largely in the area of the system Preconscious (or in the unconscious ego). Or, to put it in topographical terms, between the "two censorships" described by Freud in 1915.

II

Although we had satisfied ourselves in the Index that many of the problems surrounding the use of the term "fantasy" were related to the multiple meanings of the term, the problem of distinguishing between fantasies and theories, in particular between sexual fantasies and sexual theories, remains. In general usage, as well as in the psychoanalytic literature, the term "unconscious fantasy" is often used as a synonym for an "unconscious sexual theory," and the question arises whether it is possible and useful to distinguish between the two. Certainly, there are no clear-cut critera for distinguishing, in the material recorded in the Index, between what is a sexual fantasy and what is a sexual theory. Consider, for example, the following material derived from the analysis of a child of about 5 years of age at the time of indexing. The therapist treating the child recorded:

> Jenny quite evidently fantasied that she could achieve a fat tummy; that is, that she could become pregnant by dint of oral incorporation of food and water; and to this end she spent an inordinate amount of time compulsively consuming vast quantities of water which was often "poisonous filthy stuff" for adults, while the therapist as the baby was permitted strawberry-flavoured medicine. Water play would sometimes start as bathing the doll or cooking, but would quickly and effortlessly slide over to persistent and copious drinking during which Jenny appeared to exclude therapist and barely to relate to her. . . .
>
> During this session the child drank water poured from a toy lavatory and told the therapist she was drinking wee-wee. When later mother told the therapist that Jenny had made a comment at home that earthworms eat their own wee-wee, it seemed that an important element of her fantasy was that impregnation could occur through the drinking of urine.

We may ask: is this a fantasy or is it a theory? If it is a theory in a child of 5, what is its status if it appears in the material of an adult? Is it then a fantasy?

We have seen that a conscious daydream fantasy can be regarded as a wish-fulfilling construct of the imagination which is known by the subject not to be real. It has a certain "stamp of unreality" attached to it. But this certainly does not apply to all the thoughts which the child may have, and children have many thoughts other than fantasies. The child may come to conclusions about himself and his world, which, when looked at with adult eyes, appear to be fantasies, but have the "stamp of reality" attached to them for the child.

Freud was quite clear on the point that the fantasy is a form of thinking, and it would seem that we have a continuum between reality-appropriate thoughts on the one hand, and purely imaginative constructions, known not to be real, on the other. Of course, a great many of the thoughts of the child occupy an intermediate position between the two ends of the continuum.

In line with the discussion in the earlier part of this paper, it would appear that conscious, reality-orientated thoughts, if subsequently repressed, can later emerge in a distorted form, in one or other derivative of the Unconscious. We also know that it is highly likely that, just as we can have preconscious wish-fulfilling fantasying, so can we have preconscious reality-orientated thinking. Or, in structural terms, we can say that these processes occur in the unconscious ego.

If we return to the question of a distinction between fantasies and theories, a useful starting-off point might be the distinction that can be made in the adult between a theory and a daydream fantasy. The conscious fantasy has the hallmark of unreality, and is an imaginative production. The theory, on the other hand, is a belief about the real world which the child has created, upon which he acts, and which structures his further thinking, fantasying, and behavior. Of course, the theory may be developed on the basis of imaginative constructions, and be considered to be a derivative of instinctual wishes, but nevertheless it develops *as an explanation of reality* in contrast to the fantasy which is known to be a daydream. By starting at the conscious end, as it were, we can suggest a possible distinction between theories and fantasies. Fantasies would represent wish-fulfilling constructs of the imagination, but theories, although they may contain fantasy wish-fulfilling elements, will remain as assumptions and explanations about various aspects of the world, unless they are contradicted by reality testing. If they are contradicted, we would postulate that they do not disappear, but rather are put "out of use." In some way they can be considered to remain latent, but they can also remain operative in the construction of thoughts, ideas, and fantasies in the deeper layers of the ego (see the notion of "persistence of structures" put forward by Sandler and Joffe, 1967). The Oxford English Dictionary considers a theory to be "a systematic conception or statement of principles." It is a conception or mental scheme of something to be done, or the method of doing it, and also a statement of the rules and principles involved. It would seem that theories can be considered to be mental *structures* belonging to the whole universe of perceptual, cognitive, and logical structures which are created in order to allow the child to interpret his experience of the universe in as reality-appropriate way as possible. (That the use of such structures may be appropriate at one age, but inappropriate at another, is a separate question.) We know that careful perception will modify the child's theories,[3] but there is an interaction between theories and perception. What I am suggesting here is that the theories represent an organized part of the whole set of thinking "structures" which enter into the child's conception of the way in which the world behaves, including himself in that world, and that these structures affect not only his thinking but also memory and perception.

Before returning to the example with which this section began, it is appropriate to refer to Freud's paper (1908b) on the sexual theories of children. Freud refers to the point at which the child "comes to be occupied with the first, grand problem of life and asks himself the question: *'Where do babies come from?'*" If the child is not too intimidated, he will ask his parents directly, but usually finds that this method fails. He is generally told something like "The stork brings the babies." Freud suggests that most children are dissatisfied with such an answer, but do not always openly admit their doubts. He goes on to speak of the "further researches" of the child, usually carried out under a "cloak of secrecy." The child develops "false theories which the state of his own sexuality imposes on him." The first of these theories, says Freud, starts out from

---

[3] By the creation of further, superordinate structures, which generally also inhibit the use of the older ones.

the neglect of the differences between the sexes and consists
"in *attributing to everyone, including females, the possession of a penis,*
such as the boy knows from his own body" (p. 215). The boy's
valuation of his penis falsifies his perception, but he comes to
the conclusion that the girl's penis is too small, but when she
gets bigger it will grow. Freud then speaks of the idea of a
woman with a penis becoming "fixated" in certain individuals.
Similar theories are constructed by little girls.

Freud also points out that the second of the sexual theories
of the child is that which relates to birth. "If the baby grows in
the mother's body and is then removed from it, this can only
happen along the one possible pathway—the anal aperture. *The
baby must be evacuated like a piece of excrement, like a stool.*" Later,
further explanations are arrived at, e.g., that the baby emerges
from the navel, which opens up at birth. It follows that in both
theories of birth it is *logical* that "the child should refuse to
grant women the painful prerogative of giving birth to children" (p. 219).

The third theory referred to by Freud relates to the sadistic
view of intercourse. However, it is sufficient at this point to
emphasize that Freud spoke of children's sexual *theories,* that
even though such theories might contain wish-fulfilling elements, and be elaborated because of the pressure of particular
drives, they are felt to be *real,* and that they are used, at first
consciously, as explanations, assumptions, conclusions, and
tenets, which form the basis for the child's thinking about the
subject matter involved. One can also add to Freud's description of the child's "researches" the important factor that *the
logic of the young child differs enormously from that of the adult,* a
subject which has been studied in detail by such cognitive
psychologists as Piaget.

At this point it is worth making a further distinction which is
relevant. In the first instance, a conscious daydream fantasy, or
a conscious thought, is something *experienced* by the child. It is
located in the experiential realm of the mental apparatus (Sandler and Joffe, 1969). However, the conclusions arrived at by
the child, whether influenced by instinctual wish elements or
not, soon become "structuralized" in the nonexperiential realm.
*What was originally a thought becomes an organized and automatic
premise.* We can see this in ordinary everyday thinking about
ordinary everyday things. The theory no longer enters into the

content of the thought or fantasy, but becomes an assumption, of varying complexity, involved in the creation, in conscious or unconscious experience, of further thoughts and fantasies. The structuralized theory may be used, at a later date, to produce unconscious thought or fantasy content in the experiential realm, although such content may not be acceptable to consciousness, or allowed by the ego to proceed toward conscious experience. Nevertheless, the theory remains, as all infantile theories remain, but the products of the unconscious ego (which makes use of these theories) are either rejected, or distorted and disguised before being permitted to progress toward consciousness.

In the example quoted earlier, Jenny quite clearly had the theory that having a fat tummy was equivalent to pregnancy and that one becomes pregnant by oral incorporation of food and water. This theory colored her play, fantasies, and other derivatives, and we might expect that if she were to be in analysis as an adult, her productions would be similarly colored by her childhood theories, even though they might be much more heavily disguised.

In the construction of childhood theories, especially (but not exclusively) childhood sexual theories, we are dealing with perfectly reasonable conclusions reached by the child, using the facts at his disposal. We should take into account the fact that what is "reasonable" for a young child is not necessarily "reasonable" for an adult. The child who believes that babies are born through the anus is thinking rationally for a child of, say, 3 years of age, because he has had the experience that what appears to be a part of his body (his feces) can be separated from the body through defecation. Similarly, the child who believes in oral conception may have perfectly valid grounds at the time for believing in the reality of his theory. He may have been told that eating too much food makes one fat, that one should not eat the seeds of certain fruits (e.g., grapes) because the pips might stick in his tummy. He might also have been told that babies come from seeds, and that plants grow from seeds. He observes that when someone is to have a baby they grow fat, and so on. There are many grounds for such conclusions to be reached by the child, conclusions which are perfectly reasonable at his age, but which, if produced as theories by an older child (or by an adult) would be dismissed by himself and others as being "unreasonable." And yet in the productions of older children and of adults one sees the persistence of these earlier theories, in particular the earlier sexual theories. While a young child may consciously mention the thoughts arising on the basis of such beliefs, later such thoughts become unconscious or denied when the child knows them to be "silly," i.e., when they are subjected to reality testing they are rejected, but nevertheless still persist (Sandler and Joffe, 1967).

Implicit in this is the assumption that primitive secondary process functioning persists throughout life, although the products of such functioning can be dismissed before they reach consciousness. However, the thoughts may reappear in disguised form. It is very striking that in psychoanalytic thinking we tend to contrast primary process with secondary process functioning, but do not usually consider the contrast between one level of secondary process thinking and another.

I submit that the distinction between theories and fantasies is of clinical relevance. Indeed, we probably do make such a distinction, albeit implicitly, when we refer to unconscious fantasies. One type is the "here-and-now" fantasy: for example, a transference fantasy which may vary from one day to another. The second type, which we also tend to call "unconscious fantasies," comprises the persisting and enduring constructions which appear over and over again in the form of themes in the patient's material. The latter may well represent childhood theories which are still being invoked in the thinking that occurs in the unconscious ego. They include such theories as "all women have a penis; all fathers are castrating; anything aggressive is dangerous."

Although what has been put forward in this short account has been concerned with the well-known sexual theories of childhood, the conclusions must apply equally to all the other theories created by the developing child. The sexual theories of the child play (and have always played) an important part in psychoanalysis, but theories involving aggression, object relationships, noninstinctual factors and the like are equally important, both in child development and in the psychoanalytic reconstruction of that development.

Bibliography

ABRAHAM, K. (1916), The First Pregenital Stage of the Libido. In: *Selected Papers on Psycho-Analysis*. London: Hogarth Press, 1927, pp. 248-279.

BIBRING, E. (1953), The Mechanism of Depression. In: *Affective Disorders*, ed. P. Greenacre. New York: International Universities Press, pp. 13-48.

BONNARD, A. (1954), Some Discrepancies between Perception and Affect As Illustrated by Children in Wartime. *The Psychoanalytic Study of the Child*, 9:242-251.

BOWLBY, J. (1951), *Maternal Care and Mental Health*. Geneva; World Health Organization Monograph.

―――― (1960), Grief and Mourning in Infancy and Early Childhood. *The Psychoanalytic Study of the Child*, 15:9-52.

BRODY, S. (1970), A Mother Is Being Beaten: An Instinctual Derivative and Infant Care. In: *Parenthood: Its Psychology and Psychopathology*, ed. E. J. Anthony & T. Benedek. Boston: Little, Brown, pp. 427-447.

CREAK, M. *et al.* (1964), Schizophrenic Syndrome in Childhood. Progress Report of a Working Party. *Brit. Med. J.*, 2:889-890.

ERIKSON, E. H. (1950a), Growth and Crisis of the Healthy Personality. In: *Identity and the Life Cycle* [*Psychological Issues*, 1:50-100]. New York: International Universities Press, 1959.

―――― (1950b), *Childhood and Society*. New York: Norton.

FREUD, A. (1936), *The Ego and the Mechanisms of Defense. The Writings of Anna Freud*, Vol. 2. New York: International Universities Press, 1966.

―――― (1951), Observations on Child Development. *The Writings of Anna Freud*, 4:143-162. New York: International Universities Press, 1968.

―――― (1952), Studies in Passivity. *The Writings of Anna Freud*, 4:245-259. New York: International Universities Press, 1968.

―――― (1960), Discussion of Dr. John Bowlby's paper. *The Psychoanalytic Study of the Child*, 15:53-62.

―――― (1965a), *Normality and Pathology in Childhood. The Writings of*

Anna Freud, Vol. 6. New York: International Universities Press, 1970.

———— (1965b), Three Contributions to a Seminar on Family Law. *The Writings of Anna Freud*, 5:436-459. New York: International Universities Press, 1969.

———— (1966), Obsessional Neurosis: A Summary of Psycho-Analytic Views. *The Writings of Anna Freud*, 5:242-261. New York: International Universities Press, 1969.

———— (1968), *Indications for Child Analysis and Other Papers. The Writings of Anna Freud*, Vol. 4. New York: International Universities Press.

———— (1970), Symptomatology in Childhood: A Preliminary Attempt at Classification. *The Psychoanalytic Study of the Child*, 25:19-41.

———— & BURLINGHAM, D. (1942-43), Infants Without Families. *The Writings of Anna Freud*, Vol. 3 New York: International Universities Press, 1973.

———— NAGERA, H. & FREUD, W. E. (1965), Metapsychological Assessment of the Adult Personality: The Adult Profile. *The Psychoanalytic Study of the Child*, 20:9-41.

FREUD, S. (1907), Obsessive Actions and Religious Practices. *Standard Edition**, 9:115-127.

———— (1908a), Creative Writers and Day-Dreaming. *Standard Edition*, 9:141-153.

———— (1908b), On the Sexual Theories of Children. *Standard Edition*, 9:205-226.

———— (1911), Formulations on the Two Principles of Mental Functioning. *Standard Edition*, 12:213-226.

———— (1913), The Disposition to Obsessional Neurosis. *Standard Edition*, 12:311-326.

———— (1915), The Unconscious. *Standard Edition*, 14:159-215.

———— (1917), Mourning and Melancholia. *Standard Edition*, 14:237-260.

———— (1923), The Ego and the Id. *Standard Edition*, 19:3-66.

———— (1924), The Economic Problem of Masochism. *Standard Edition*, 19:157-170.

———— (1926), Inhibitions, Symptoms and Anxiety. *Standard Edition*, 20:77-175.

———— (1950), *The Origins of Psychoanalysis: Letters, Drafts and Notes to Wilhelm Fliess (1887-1902)*, New York: Basic Books, 1954, p. 196.

* *The Standard Edition of the Complete Psychological Works of Sigmund Freud*, 23 Volumes. London: Hogarth Press, 1953-1966.

GOLDSTEIN, J., FREUD, A., & SOLNIT, A. J. (1973), *Beyond the Best Interests of the Child.* New York: Free Press.
—— & KATZ, J. (1962), Invitation to Dr. Anna Freud. (Unpublished memo to Dean Eugene Rostow, dated 2nd January 1962.)
—— —— (1965), *The Family and the Law.* New York: Free Press, pp. 1051-1053.
GREENACRE, P. (1923), A Study of the Mechanism of Obsessive-Compulsive Conditions. *Amer. J. Psychiat.*, 2:527-538.
—— (1968), Perversions: General Considerations Regarding Their Genetic and Dynamic Background. *The Psychoanalytic Study of the Child*, 23:47-62.
HARTMANN, H. (1939), *Ego Psychology and the Problem of Adaptation.* New York: International Universities Press, 1958.
HOFFER, W. (1950), Oral Aggressiveness and Ego Development. *Int. J. Psycho-Anal.*, 31:156-160.
JACOBSON, E. (1965), A Special Response to Early Object Loss. *Depression.* New York: International Universities Press, 1971, pp. 185-203.
—— (1971), *Depression.* New York: International Universities Press.
JOFFE, W. G. & SANDLER, J. (1965), Notes on Pain, Depression, and Individuation. *The Psychoanalytic Study of the Child*, 20:394-424.
KOHUT, H. (1971), *The Analysis of the Self.* New York: International Universities Press.
KRIS, E. (1947), The Nature of Psychoanalytic Propositions and Their Validation. In: *Freedom and Experience*, ed. S. Hook & M. R. Konwitz. Ithaca, N. Y.: Cornell University Press, pp. 239-259.
LEWIN, B. D. (1948), The Neuroses and Their Accompaniment in Physical Dysfunction. In: *Synopsis of Psychosomatic Diagnosis and Treatment*, ed. F. Dunbar. St. Louis: C. V. Mosby, pp. 398-408.
LUSTMAN, S. L. (1967), The Scientific Leadership of Anna Freud. *J. Amer. Psychoanal. Assn.*, 15:810-827.
MAHLER, M. S. (1961), On Sadness and Grief in Infancy and Childhood: Loss and Restoration of the Symbiotic Love Object. *The Psychoanalytic Study of the Child*, 16:332-351.
—— (1968), *On Human Symbiosis and the Vicissitudes of Individuation, Volume 1: Infantile Psychosis.* New York: International Universities Press.
—— (1971), A Study of the Separation-Individuation Process. *The Psychoanalytic Study of the Child*, 26:403-424.
NAGERA, H. (1965), On Obsessional Neurosis. Unpublished manuscript.
NOVICK, J. & HURRY, A. (1969), Projection and Externalization. *J. Child Psychotherapy*, 2:5-20.

RADFORD, P., WISEBERG, S. & YORKE, C. (1972), A Study of "Main-Line" Heroin Addiction: A Preliminary Report. *The Psychoanalytic Study of the Child*, 27:156-180.

ROSENFELD, S. & SPRINCE, M. P. (1963), An Attempt to Formulate the Meaning of the Concept "Borderline." *The Psychoanalytic Study of the Child*, 18:603-635.

——— ——— (1965), Some Thoughts on the Technical Handling of Borderline Children. *The Psychoanalytic Study of the Child*, 20:495-517.

RUBINFINE, D. L. (1962), Maternal Stimulation, Psychic Structure, and Early Object Relations: With Special Reference to Aggression and Denial. *The Psychoanalytic Study of the Child*, 17:265-282.

SANDLER, J. (1962), The Hampstead Index as an Instrument of Psycho-Analytic Research. *Int. J. Psycho-Anal.*, 43:289-291.

——— & JOFFE, W. G. (1967), The Tendency to Persistence In Psychological Function and Development With Special Reference to the Processes of Fixation and Regression. *Bull. Menninger Clin.*, 31:257.

——— ——— (1969), Towards a Basic Psychoanalytic Model. *Int. J. Psycho-Anal.*, 50:79-90.

——— & NAGERA, H. (1963), Aspects of the Metapsychology of Fantasy. *The Psychoanalytic Study of the Child*, 18:159-194.

——— NOVICK, J., & YORKE, C. (1970), The Hampstead Child-Therapy Course and Clinic, London.

SCHAFER, R. (1968), *Aspects of Internalization*. New York: International Universities Press.

SEARLES, H. F. (1969), A Case of Borderline Thought Disorder. *Int. J. Psycho-anal.*, 50:655-664.

SPITZ, R. A. & WOLF, K. M. (1946), Anaclitic Depression: An Inquiry into the Genesis of Psychiatric Conditions in Early Childhood, II. *The Psychoanalytic Study of the Child*, 2:313-342.

SYLVESTER, E. (1947), Pathogenic Influences of Maternal Attitudes in the Neonatal Period. *Problems of Early Infancy*, ed. M. J. Senn. New York: J. Macy, Jr. Foundation, pp. 67-70.

——— (1954), Developmental Truisms and Their Fate in Child Rearing. *Problems of Infancy and Early Childhood*, ed. M. J. Senn. New York: J. Macy, Jr. Foundation, pp. 9-37.

THOMAS, R. ET AL. (1966), Comments on Some Aspects of Self and Object Representation in a Group of Psychotic Children: An Application of Anna Freud's Diagnostic Profile. *The Psychoanalytic Study of the Child*, 21:527-580.

WINNICOTT, D. W. (1958), *Collected Papers*. New York: Basic Books.

WOLFENSTEIN, M. (1966), How Is Mourning Possible? *The Psychoanalytic Study of the Child,* 21:93-123.

YORKE, C. (1970), A Critical Review of Some Psycho-Analytic Literature on Drug Addiction. *Brit. J. Med. Psychol.,* 43:141-159.

—— DAVIDSON, A., & ISAACS, S. (1970), Memorandum for the Home Office, Departmental Committee on Adoption under the Chairmanship of Sir William Houghton. London: The British Psycho-Analytical Society.

Program for the Twentieth Anniversary Celebrations of the Hampstead Clinic

OPENING ADDRESSES

ANNA FREUD
ALBERT J. SOLNIT
JOSEPH GOLDSTEIN

CLINICAL PRESENTATIONS

Reflections on Borderline and Atypical Cases: Borderline Functioning in a Traumatized Atypical Child
SARA ROSENFELD (*Study Group for Borderline Cases*)

Depressive Phenomena in Childhood: Their Open and Disguised Manifestations in Analytic Treatment
AGNES BENE (*Technique Group*)

A Report on the Analysis of a 15-Year-Old Boy with Severe Sadomasochistic Fixations
HANNA KENNEDY

Simultaneous Analysis of Parents and Children
ILSE HELLMAN

Problems over Identification in a Partially Sighted Child
MARIA KAWENOKA BERGER

An Interdisciplinary Approach to the Sick Child and His Family
BIANCA GORDON

The Border between Therapy and Education
ROSE EDGCUMBE

Some War Babies Thirty Years Later: Follow-up Report
ILSE HELLMAN

170

DIAGNOSTIC STUDIES

Some Problems of Diagnosis in Children Presenting with Obsessional Symptomatology
   CLIFFORD YORKE (*Study Group for Diagnostic Assessment*)

Some Preliminary Findings in a Systematic Research Project
   PATRICIA RADFORD, STANLEY WISEBERG, AND CLIFFORD YORKE (*Study Group of "Mainline" Heroin Addiction*)

The Use of the Profile Schema for the Psychotic Patient
   THOMAS FREEMAN (*Study Group of Adult Psychoses*)

INDEX STUDIES

Sexual Fantasies and Sexual Theories in Childhood
   JOSEPH SANDLER (*Index Research Group*)

A General Outline of the Index Research Project
   JOSEPH SANDLER (*and members of the Index Group*)

DEVELOPMENT OF BLIND CHILDREN

Film presentations: "Growing Up Without Sight" and "Nursery School for the Blind"
   DOROTHY BURLINGHAM (*Study Group of the Development of Blind Children*)

PLENARY SESSION

Symposium on Training at Hampstead
   Contributions by RUTH THOMAS, I. ELKAN, AND A STUDENT REPRESENTATIVE
   Discussion by ANNA FREUD AND HEADS OF STUDY GROUPS

Glimpses of Historical Films

CLOSING REMARKS

   K. R. EISSLER
   ANNA FREUD

Index

Abraham, K., 35, 163
Accidents, 8-13, 50, 58-59
Addiction, "mainline," 99-116
Adolescence, 34, 39, 44
  and onset of obessional neurosis, 93
  and drug addiction, 109, 116
Adoption
  common-law, 24-28
  contested, 18-29
Affect
  depressive, 33, 36, 44
  and fantasy, 150-54
Aggression
  anal, 95-96
  in borderline child, 56, 58-62
  and depression, 35-36, 42-43
  fear of, 77
  inhibition of, 77, 93, 110-11
  and obsessional symptoms, 82-97
  and pain, 58
  in psychosis, 118, 121-22
  and self-esteem regulation, 104,
    106-07, 114, 116
  turned against self, 56-57
  see also Identification with aggres-
    sor, Rage
Alcoholism, 92, 101
Ambivalence and depression, 36, 44
Anxiety
  in borderline children, 50-62
  of parents, 95
  in psychosis, 121, 125
  see also Fear
Anxiety-proneness, 67
Art, 153, 156
Assessment, see Diagnosis, Profile
Autoerotism in borderline child, 50,
  60-62

Bar Mitzvah and symptom formation,
  83-85, 88, 91
Battered child, 7

Beating of child, 58
Behavior
  antisocial and psychotic, 48
  observation of, 2-8; see also Direct
    observation
  sadomasochistic, 34, 36, 41
Bene, A., vii, 33-46
Berger, M. K., 65-80
Bibring, E., 35-36, 163
Blind children, 7
  analysis of, 65-80
Bond, D. D., vii
Bonnard, A., 48, 163
Borderline cases, 144
  treatment of, 47-63
Bowlby, J., 23, 43, 163
Brody, S., 58, 163
Burlingham, D., ix, 1, 15, 17, 163,
  164

Castration anxiety and blindness, 68,
  73
Chapsky v. Wood, 28
Character, oral, 115
Child
  developmental needs of, 127
  disadvantaged, 4, 127-32, 135-47
  management of severely injured,
    8-13
  need to protect mother, 91-93,
    96-97
  playing fool, 44
  right to be wanted, 24-29
  sexual theories of, 149-62
  taking on mother's illness, 91-93,
    96-97
  underprivileged, 127-32, 135-47
Child advocate, 13
Child analysis
  compared to adult analysis, x-xii,
    42
  developments in, 1-13
  and education, 134-47

follow-up, 39-40
of narcissistic disturbances, 42-46
technical problems with depressive
phenomena, 33-46
technique, xi-xii
Child placement, 16, 29
least detrimental alternative, 24-27
Childhood psychosis, 125
Compulsion to repeat, 51
Conflict
bisexual in blind boy, 70-80
internalized, 138-46
in psychosis, 119
somatic dramatization, 89
Consciousness, 2, 151-62
Conversion hysteria, 89
Creak, M., 125, 163
Currier, Mrs., vii

Davidson, A., 23, 167
Day care, 4
Daydream, 149-60
Death wishes, 77, 97
Defense
against anal drive, 88
analysis, 42, 98
and depressive phenomena, 34-46
against dirt, 96
obsessional, 97-98
in psychosis, 118, 124
Delusion, 122-24, 150, 152, 156
Denial
of affect, 68-69, 79
and depression, 34, 37, 41
Dependence on object world, 83,
94-95
Depression (in adults), 33-36
Depressive phenomena in childhood,
33-46
Development
delayed, 133-48
normal, x-xi, 133-35
sources of knowledge about, x-xii,
2-8
Developmental lines, xi
Diagnosis, xi-xii
of children with obsessional symptoms, 81-98
of disadvantaged children, 136-37
Direct observation, 2-8; *see also* Behavior
Dirt, preoccupation with, 82-83,
86-96

Disappointment, 33-44
Displacement, 90-91
Dramatization, 89, 149
Drawing, of child going blind, 65-80
Dreams, 150, 153

Edgcumbe, R., 133-47
Education and therapy, border between, 133-47; *see also* Nursery
school
Ego
in borderline children, 48-61
delayed development, 133-47
and depression, 35-36
and education, 133-47
and fantasy, 155-62
immaturity of child's, 43
and obsessional symptomatology,
83, 96
precocious development, 82, 92
in psychosis, 118-19, 124-25
Eissler, K. R., vii
Encopresis, 84-85
Enuresis, 91
Environment, "good enough," 48, 50,
59
Epinosic gain, 95
Erikson, E. H., 27, 163
Evans, R., 61
Externalization, 49-50, 52, 60, 122,
124, 143

Family advocate, 13
Family law, 17-18
Family romance, 71
Fantasy
in borderline children, 48, 51-60
of blind children, 66-80
sexual, in children, 149-62
themes, 150
unconscious, 149-62
Fear
of contamination, 92, 97
of loss of identity, 125
see also Anxiety
Fleck, S., 49
Fliess, W., 151
Freeman, T., 117-26
Freud, A., vii-xii, 1-5, 15-18, 23, 43,
45, 62, 81-82, 95, 98, 99, 119,
125, 127-32, 133, 163-65
Freud, S., 35, 58, 93-94, 98, 150-54,
156, 158-60, 164

Freud, W. E., 119, 164
Friedlaender, K., ix
Friedman, A., 135, 138, 142

Goldberg, S., 15
Goldstein, J., 15-29, 165
Greenacre, P., 58, 93, 165
Greenson, R. R., viii, 97

Hahn, M., vii
Hallucination, 150
Hampstead Child-Therapy Course
    and Clinic, 2-4, 6-8, 13, 15, 18,
    20, 23, 28-29
  Clinical Services, 7, 65
  Concept Study Group, xi, 7
  definition of tasks of, ix
  Diagnostic Services, 7, 132
  Education Unit, 129, 133; *see also*
    Nursery School
  Group for the Study of: Adult
    Psychosis, 7, 117; Borderline
    Cases, 7, 47; Diagnostic As-
    sessment, 81; "Mainline"
    Addiction, 99; Technical
    Problems, 7, 33
  Index Research Group, xi, 7, 149
  Nursery School for Blind, xii, 7
  Profile Study Group, 7
  War Nurseries, ix, 1-2, 4
  Well-Baby Clinic, 7
Hand-washing compulsion, 83, 86-91,
    96
Hartmann, H., 50, 165
Hazen, L., viii
Helplessness, 35-36, 42, 44
Heroin addiction, 99-116
Hoffer, W., 56, 165
Hurry, A., 60, 165
Hypochondriasis, 91-93, 96-97, 123
Hypnagogic phenomena, 156
Hypomania, 44

Identification, 42-43, 45
  with aggressor, 48, 53, 62, 145-46
  in borderline children, 52-57
  and merging, 48
  primitive, 125
Incorporation, oral, 157, 161
Integrative function, 48, 54
Intellectualization, 82, 89, 93
Interpretation with borderline chil-
    dren, 54-56, 60

Isaacs, S., 23, 167

Jackson, E., 1
Jacobson, E., 35, 165
Joffe, W. G., 35, 159, 160, 162, 165,
    166

Katz, J., 15, 17, 165
Kohut, H., 36, 41, 43, 165
Kris, E., 3-5, 165

Latency and onset of obsessional
    neurosis, 93-94
Law and child placement, 16-29
Lewin, B. D., 93, 165
Libido
  and addiction, 103, 107-08, 111
  in psychosis, 117-25
Lustman, S. L., 15, 165

Mahler, M. S., 35-36, 49, 59, 165
Masturbation, 75
  and addiction, 103-04
Memory and fantasy, 150-62
Merging, 48, 125
Mood in psychosis, 124
Morrison, A., vii
Mother, impact of child on, 90
Mothering, inconsistent, 58-59
Mother-child relationship
  and borderline cases, 47-49, 58-59
  early, 40-41, 43
  sadomasochistic, 144-46
  see also Parent
Mother guidance, 145
Motility, disturbed in psychosis,
    122-24

Nagera, H., 94, 119, 149, 152, 155,
    164, 165, 166
Narcissism
  and addiction, 99, 103, 107, 116
  premature frustration, 41-46
Narcissistic disturbances and depres-
    sive phenomena, 33-46
Negativism, 123-24
Neurosis, obsessional (adult), 81-98
Nightmare, 101
Novick, J., 7, 60, 165, 166
Nunberg, H., vii
Nursery School (of Hampstead
    Child-Therapy Course and
    Clinic), 4, 7, 127-32, 135-47

for blind, xii, 7
influence on family life, 132
physical care in, 129-30, 141
promoting verbalization, 130-31
as source of stimulation and experience, 131-32, 138-40
as substitute parent, 130
tasks, 128-29

Object, used for defensive purposes, 98
Object choice, 123
Object loss and depression, 34, 43
Object relations
and addiction, 103-04
of borderline children, 47-63
delayed development, 133-47
in obsessional children, 88-98
Object representation in borderline children, 49, 59-63
Obsessional symptomatology in children, 81-98
Oedipal phase, 38-39, 43-44, 87
Operations, 72-76, 85

Painting, 149; see also Drawing
Paranoia, 120, 124
Parent
abandoning child, 19-29
blind, 65-78
collaborating with pediatricians, 10-13
colluding with child, 95
deaf-mute, 45
fear of child's temper tantrum, 95
pathology of, 144-46
psychological, 23-29
see also Mother-child relationship
Passivity, defensive, 142-43
Penis, illusory, 159-62
Penis envy, 103
and depression, 34, 37-38, 41
Perception, 155, 159-60
Physical handicap, 4, 7-8, 86, 90; see also Blind children
Phobia, 91-92
Piaget, J., 160
Preconscious, 150-53
Profile
for addict, 99-100
developmental, 7-8, 133

diagnostic, xi, 97, 119-20
for psychotic patients, 117-26
Projection, 49-50, 60, 122, 124-25, 143
Promiscuity, 102-04
Protest, 43
Psychoanalysis, applications of, xii, 7-13, 15-18
Psychoanalytic training, ix, xii, 4, 6
"ideal" case, 45
Psychoanalytic Index, xi, 149
Psychosis, 117-26
adult and childhood compared, 125-26
course and outcome, 120-23
symptomatology and classification, 123-25
Puberty, see Adolescence
Putzel, R., 81-98

Radford, P., 99-116, 166
Rage, 50, 56
Reality, psychic, 152-53
Reality testing
in borderline children, 58-60
and fantasy, 151-62
Regression
and obsessional defenses, 97
and progression, 44-45
in psychosis, 123-24
Remedial work, 138-47
Repression and fantasy, 150, 156-58
Research, psychoanalytic, 4-8, 125-26
microscopic and macroscopic approach, 5-6
Rosenfeld, S., 47-63, 166
Ross, H., vii, 51
Rostow, E., 16
Rubinfine, D., 36, 166
Rumination, 89

Sadism, 95
Safety, area of, 52-58
Sandler, J., 7, 35, 149-62, 165, 166
Schacht, L., 81-98
Schafer, R., 49, 52, 166
Schizophrenia, 124; see also Psychosis
Searles, H. F., 48, 166
Self
cohesive, 48, 59, 61
development, 41, 61
and hand-mouth coordination, 56

Self-attack, 106
Self cathexis, in heroin addict, 99-116
Self-esteem
  and addiction, 103-116
  and depression, 33-46
Self-object differentiation, 48, 51, 60
Self representation in borderline
  children, 48-49, 53, 59-63
Senn, M. J. E., 166
Separation-individuation, 49, 59
Sexuality, childhood fantasies and
  theories of, 149-62
Shapira, A., 15
Sibling rivalry, 68-69, 137-38
Signal anxiety, 61
Sleep disturbances, 101
Solnit, A. J., 1-13, 18, 165
Speech disturbances, 125
Spitz, R. A., 35, 43, 166
Sprince, M., 47, 166
Sublimation, 42-43, 45, 133
  dearth of, 93
Superego
  and depression, 44
  and obsessional children, 83, 90
  in psychosis, 118, 142
Sylvester, E., 61, 166
Symbolization, 82, 91, 93
Symptom
  classification of psychotic, 123-25
  and fantasy, 153
  formation and separation, 88
  obsessional, *see* Obsessional symp-
    tomatology
Synthetic function, 116

TAT, 85, 95
Teacher and therapist, 134-35
Temper tantrum, 95, 101, 131,
  141-42
Testicle, undescended, 85
Thomas, R., 47, 51, 61, 125, 166
Thought processes
  and fantasy, 150-62
  in psychosis, 125-26
Toilet training, 38
Transference
  in borderline children, 52, 59-60
  in child analysis, 42
  and defense, 98
  fantasy, 149, 156, 162
Transitional object, 103
Trauma
  narcissistic, 33-44
  ongoing, 47-62
Treatment alliance, 98

Unconscious, 152-62

Verbalization, promotion of, 130-31,
  139-47

Winnicott, D. W., 48, 50, 59, 166
Wiseberg, S., 99-116, 166
Wish and fantasy, 150-58
Wolf, K. M., 35, 43, 166
Wolfenstein, M., 43, 167

Yale University
  Child Study Center, xii, 1
  Law School, xii, 15-17
Yorke, C., 7, 23, 81-116, 166, 167